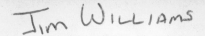

PLYOMETRICS

Explosive Power Training

Second Edition

James C. Radcliffe, BS
Robert C. Farentinos, PhD

Human Kinetics Publishers, Inc.
Champaign, Illinois

Library of Congress Cataloging-in-Publication Data

Radcliffe, James C. (James Christopher), 1958-
   Plyometrics : explosive power training.

   Bibliography: p.
   1. Physical education and training.   2. Exercise.
3. Exercise—Physiological aspects.   I. Farentinos,
Robert C., 1941-   II. Title.
GV711.5.R33   1985   613.7′1   85-14409
ISBN 0-87322-024-2

Editor: Peg Goyette
Production director: Sara Chilton
Typesetter: Sandra Meier
Text layout: Lezli Harris
Illustrator: Mary Yemma Long
Muscle illustrations (page 8): Gail A. Irwin
Cover design: Julie Szamocki
Printed by: United Graphics, Inc.

ISBN: 0-87322-024-2

Printed in the United States of America

10 9 8 7 6 5 4 3 2

Human Kinetics Publishers, Inc.
Box 5076
Champaign, Illinois 61820

To our parents for their ever-present
support and encouragement

CONTENTS

PREFACE

During the past 2 years we have conducted an extensive program of plyometric training involving a variety of athletes and fitness enthusiasts. Our subjects have included professional football players, cross-country skiers (two of whom participated in the 1984 Olympics), marathon and mountain runners, weightlifters, basketball players, young athletes, and older fitness buffs. The list includes many members of the Farentinos Gym, a training and conditioning facility that we operate in Boulder, Colorado.

One of us, Jim, has a practical background in plyometrics that spans almost a decade. Most of the drills presented in this book are his creation, the result of much research and coaching in this area. In fact, this book is a direct outcome of Jim's original book, *Plyometrics Methods Notebook*, published in 1983.

The other, Bob, a former competitive weightlifter, is now a member of the U.S. Marathon Ski Team. In this book Bob applies his considerable knowledge of anatomy and biology to plyometric training, and in turn uses this knowledge of plyometrics to enhance his own training for Nordic skiing.

We wrote this book for coaches and athletes who wish to know more about plyometrics and how to apply this dynamic training method to specific sports. We also produced a 50-minute videotape to complement this book. (See page 129 for information about purchasing the tape from the publisher.)

We are deeply committed to plyometric training and use it daily in our own workouts and in directing the training of others. We also have reviewed all the research we could find on plyometrics, and present these findings along with our own experiences. Our objective in this book is to provide a more systematic and comprehensive treatment of plyometrics than has been offered before. It is intended to be a practical, "how to" book.

The book is organized into three parts. Part I defines plyometrics, presents a brief history, and describes the principles of how and why plyometrics works. In Part II you will learn about how plyometrics enhances the movements required to perform skillfully in sports. We also present in Part II the basic principles for executing plyometric exercises. In Part III we describe and illustrate 40 plyometric exercises which can be used for specific athletic activities. The Appendix contains a more technical discussion about the physiological basis of plyometric exercises.

This second edition contains more information on the testing and use of plyometric techniques. Instead of photographs, you will find line drawings made from photo sequences to better illustrate the plyometric exercises.

We are grateful to a number of people who helped us with this book: certainly all of the members at Farentinos Gym who so willingly did their "plyos," and all the coaches, especially Mike Lopez, who worked with Jim Radcliffe over the years and listened to his preaching and postulation about the virtues of plyometric training. We received valuable assistance from Greg Bezer, Harvey Newton, Ed Burke, Don Nielsen, Audun Endestad, Pat Ahern, Dave Felkley, Dan Allen, Steve Ilg, John Tansley, Rick Johnson, I.J. Gorman, Steven Farentinos, and others as well.

We have enjoyed the personal and professional associations with all concerned and truly hope we have returned the favor in some way.

James C. Radcliffe
and Robert C. Farentinos
Boulder, Colorado

Part I UNDERSTANDING PLYOMETRICS

Plyometrics is a method of developing explosive power, an important component of most athletic performances. From a practical point of view plyometric training is relatively easy to teach and learn, and it places fewer physical demands on the body than strength or endurance training. Plyometrics rapidly is becoming an integral part of the overall training program in many sports.

From a physiological perspective, plyometrics is perplexing. Practical experience supports its value, yet we do not fully understand how it works. Although some of the basic neuromuscular processes underlying plyometrics are known, little research has been done on what actually occurs at this level as a result of plyometric training.

In Part I you will learn what plyometrics means and take a brief look at its history. Then you will learn the basic principles of plyometric training.

Chapter 1 WHAT ARE PLYOMETRIC EXERCISES?

PLYOMETRICS DEFINED

Beginning with the ancient Greeks, coaches and athletes have sought methods and techniques for improving speed and strength. Speed and strength combined is power, and power is essential in performing most sport skills, whether the tennis serve or the clean and jerk. Although specific exercises designed to enhance quick, explosive movements have been taught for some time, only in the last decade has a system emerged which emphasizes "explosive-reactive" power training. This new system of athletic training is known as plyometrics.

The origin of the term *plyometrics* is thought to be derived from the Greek word "pleythyein," meaning to augment or to increase, or from the Greek root words "plio" and "metric," mean-

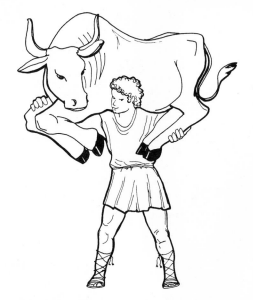

ing more and measure, respectively (Chu, 1983; Gambetta, 1981; Wilt & Ecker, 1970). Today plyometrics refers to exercises characterized by powerful muscular contractions in response to

rapid, dynamic loading or stretching of the involved muscles.

Plyometric movements are performed in a wide spectrum of sports in which power is useful. For example, consider the football lineman coming out of the stance, the volleyball player jumping up high above the net to block the return, the high jumper at take-off, and the baseball batter swinging at a pitch. The basketball player shooting the ball and then quickly jumping back up to get the rebound or tip-in can benefit from plyometrics. The platform diver who needs more height at the take-off can enhance performance through plyometrics. The tennis player or the baseball outfielder who needs to move more quickly to the ball to make the play will also benefit from plyometric training. Most sports can be played more skillfully when athletes have the power that combines strength and speed. Plyometrics is one of the best ways to develop explosive power for sports.

HISTORY OF PLYOMETRICS

The modern history of plyometric training is brief. Its impetus and recognition as a useful technique for increasing explosive power came primarily from the Russian and Eastern European successes in track and field beginning in the mid-1960s. An early proponent of plyometrics was Yuri Veroshanski, the Russian coach whose accomplishments with jumpers is legendary. Veroshanski (1967) experimented with depth jumps and the shock method as plyometric techniques for increasing his athletes' reactive ability. An important aspect of Veroshanski's conceptualization of plyometrics was his contention that plyometric training helped develop the whole neuromuscular system for power

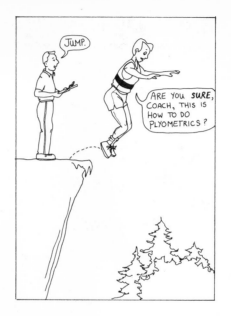

movements, not merely the contractile tissue alone.

Plyometrics received a big boost from the remarkable performances of the Russian sprinter Valeri Borzov, who credited much of his success to plyometric training. In the 1972 Olympic Games, at the age of 20, Borzov won the 100-meter event in 10.0 seconds.

The astonishing thing about Borzov's achievement was that 6 years earlier his 100-meter times had hovered around 13 seconds, which did not indicate potential world-class capabilities. The increase in Borzov's sprinting prowess was largely due to his physiological maturation from the age of 14 to 20, but his success also has been attributed to the rigorous plyometric training he undertook throughout this period.

PLYOMETRICS TODAY

The stories told in gymnasiums and on training fields about plyometrics tend to enshrine this form of training. For example, an Olympic weightlifter who weighed over 300 lbs. is reported to have jumped from a flat-footed position on the floor onto a platform located at his eye-level height. The credit for this feat is given to plyometric training.

In this book we do not want to

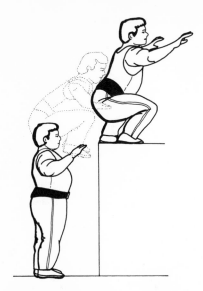

John Tansley, Dwight Stones's coach during some of his best years, states that Stones was not exceptionally strong and did not have great speed; furthermore, he had relatively poor jumping ability when tested in the vertical jump. Yet he outjumped everybody else. Tansley believes Stones's work with plyometrics had a good deal to do with it.

Plyometric exercises are helping athletes in football, basketball, soccer, weightlifting, swimming, Nordic and Alpine skiing, baseball and other sports. Any sport skill demanding power—the combination of speed and strength—can benefit from plyometric training.

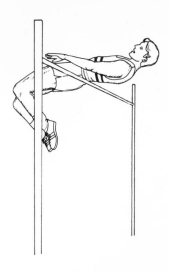

embellish plyometric training with magical qualities; it does not permit athletes to perform superhuman feats. But we do want you to know that plyometric training has gained worldwide acceptance and credibility through scientific research (Bosco & Komi, 1979, 1981; Chu, 1983; Gambetta, 1981; Wilt & Ecker, 1970) and true success stories such as the "Fosbury Flop" (Tansley, 1980).

Chapter 2 PLYOMETRIC BASICS

Useful analogies can be made between the structural elements of the human body and the mechanics of support systems as described by the engineer. Elasticity, strength, loading, compression, and tension are properties not only of concrete and steel but also of bone cartilage, tendons, and ligaments. Thus, the mandible can be likened to an I-beam girder and the zygomatic arch to a floor joist, or the load characteristics of the femur can be compared with those of a concrete column. Similarly, descriptions of human movements as they occur in sports can be better understood using the concepts of force, work, acceleration, velocities, levers, and torques. And in the same way, analogies can be made between systems that control motor skills and electronic relay systems, servo-mechanisms, and computers.

In our analysis and application of plyometrics, we use various models, comparisons, and terminologies borrowed from the world of machines and electronics. We do this to help elucidate, but with the awareness that actual performance of human athletic skills never occurs as merely the sum of such factors as strength, velocity, loading, and stretch. Actual performance of any movement pattern, plyometric or otherwise, is holistic in nature, a total integration of all such factors. In the development and use of human power, the volitional (mind) mechanisms that drive and coordinate the skeletal musculature may be even more important than the muscle fiber itself. Enhancement of muscular control and reactive power associated with plyometric exercise apparently is related to changes in complex neuromuscular structure and sensory-motor pathways.

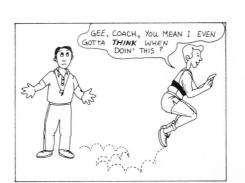

HOW PLYOMETRIC TRAINING WORKS

The basis of both the voluntary and involuntary motor processes involved in plyometrics is the so-called "stretch reflex," which is also called the muscle spindle reflex or myotatic reflex. This spindle apparatus and the stretch reflex are vital components of the nervous system's overall control of body movement. In the execution of many learned athletic skills just prior to an explosive-reactive movement, the muscles may undergo a rapid stretching as a result of some type of load placed upon them. Such a "cocking-phase" (Chu, 1983) occurs in the hitting of a baseball or swinging of a golf club. What is being accomplished by the batter or golfer unknowingly during this cocking phase is a rapid

but slight lengthening of muscle fibers in those muscle groups responsible for generating the power of the swing. The rapid stretching (loading) of these muscles activates the muscle spindle reflex which sends a very strong stimulus via the spinal cord to the muscles, causing them to contract powerfully.

For example, when the right-handed golfer shown below begins the backswing, the bicep muscle of the left arm contracts and the tricep is stretched.

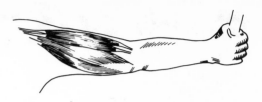

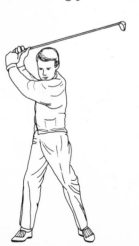

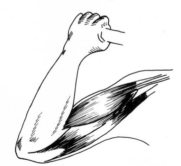

Then when the golfer begins the forward swing, as shown above, the tricep contracts powerfully in response to its rapid stretching which activated the muscle spindle reflex.

Various terms have been suggested to describe phases of the stretch reflex. Chu (1983) referred to the rapid loading of the muscle fibers immediately prior to muscle contraction as the "eccentric phase," the brief period of time between initiation of the eccentric phase and the reflex muscle contraction as the "amortization phase," and contraction itself as the "concentric phase." Veroshanski (1967) has labeled the loading or stretching of the muscle fibers the "yielding phase" and the ensuing reflex contraction the "overcoming phase," as shown above. We find Veroshanski's terminology more helpful in teaching plyometrics.

Plyometric exercises are thought to stimulate various changes in the neuromuscular system, enhancing the ability of the muscle groups to respond more quickly and powerfully to slight and rapid changes in muscle length. An important feature of plyometric training apparently is the conditioning of the neuromuscular system to allow for faster and more powerful changes of direction, for example, going from down to up in jumping or moving the legs first anteriorly then posteriorly in running. Reducing the time needed for this change in direction increases speed and power.

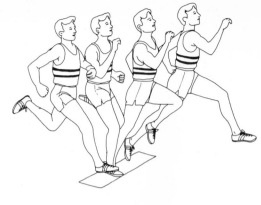

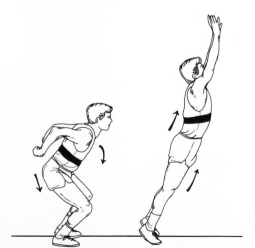

This is but a basic explanation of how plyometric training works. If you would like to learn more about the physiological and neurological processes thought to be involved in plyometrics, you will find a detailed explanation of them in Appendix A.

PRINCIPLES OF ATHLETIC TRAINING

Certain principles of athletic training applicable to other forms of exercise

also apply to plyometrics. One of the most basic and widely accepted is the progressive overload principle, which has been employed with great success in developing strength, power, and endurance. The relationship between increasing muscular strength and resistive overload using weights is quite well known. Repetition of a work load that is less than an overload emphasizes endurance of the muscle, not its strength.

Because the emphasis is on power development in plyometrics, and because power is defined as strength and frequency or strength divided by time, both resistive and temporal overloads must be applied. In plyometric exercise, resistive overloads usually take the form of a rapid change of direction of a limb or the entire body, such as overcoming the increased g-forces as the result of falling, stepping, bounding, hopping, leaping, or jumping. For example, as shown on page 10, the overload is increased by the athlete falling from progressively higher plat-

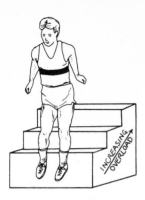

durance. Furthermore, development of aerobic power and muscular strength for cross-country skiing, bicycling, or running can most effectively be accomplished when training is focused on the specific muscle groups used in each of these sports. Specific exercise elicits specific adaptations, thus creating specific training effects (McArdle, Katch, & Katch, 1981).

The principle of specificity also applies in plyometric exercise. Some plyometric movements are designed to enhance striding power, others are used to increase jumping ability, and still others may specifically work the twisting muscles of the torso. The application of specific plyometric exercises is determined by the athlete's own desired performance goal.

In addition to the concepts of resistive (amounts and distances) and temporal (time and intensity) overload, it is useful to conceptualize an overload system based on the spatial dimension. That is, movements can also have the effects of overload from

the standpoint of range of motion. The concept is to employ the stretch reflex within a specific range of motion. If the range of motion is too great, then the purpose is defeated because of failure to initiate a reflexive action. However, many plyometric exercises—although specific to particular athletic skills in terms of plane of movement of limbs and involvement of certain muscle groups—are executed in a spatially exaggerated manner; that is, limbs may be carried through much wider ranges of motion even though the actual plane of movement resembles that of the performance goal.

The pole-bounding exercise of cross-country skiers, for example, requires that the exerciser simulate the diagonal stride of skiing but that the range of contralateral motion of arms and legs be somewhat exaggerated to maximize intensity of the movement. Thus, the specific plyometric effect is achieved not only by overloads working at the resistive and temporal levels but also at the spatial levels. Resistive,

forms. A temporal overload can be accomplished by concentrating on executing the movement as rapidly and intensely as possible.

Another general tenet of athletic training is the principle of specificity. In the context of athletic training, specificity refers to neuromuscular and metabolic adaptations of particular systems in response to particular types of overload. Exercise stress such as strength training for certain muscle groups induces specific strength adaptations in these muscle groups; increases in endurance can only be achieved effectively by training for en-

temporal, and spatial overload are important considerations, as are specificity and training frequency, intensity, and duration, topics more fully discussed in Parts II and III.

Part II TRAINING MOVEMENTS AND METHODS

A wide variety of movements and action sequences are seen in sports. Some are quite simple and involve relatively few learned skill components, but others are exceedingly complicated. Similarly, in plyometric training a broad spectrum of simple to complex exercises is available. Deciding which to use depends upon your particular athletic performance goals.

In Part II we introduce a system for categorizing plyometric exercises based upon functional anatomy and its relationship with athletic movement. Thus, the exercises can be separated on the basis of the musculature involved and how it relates to particular sport movements. We examine the major muscle groups involved in movements basic to many sports and provide a rationale for using certain drills to train that muscle group to perform the movement more powerfully.

Next we present the guidelines to follow for efficient development of explosive power. Proper execution of plyometric exercises is vital for achieving the maximum benefits of this form of training and for avoiding injury.

Chapter 3 MOVEMENTS AND MUSCLE GROUPS

Various plyometric exercises are described and illustrated in Part III. These exercises are organized according to three basic muscle groups: (a) legs and hips, (b) midsection or trunk, and (c) chest, shoulder girdle, and arms. Although considered separately here, these three categories are functionally integrated; they are parts of the human "power chain" (Landis, 1983).

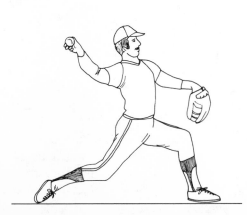

Most athletic movement originates from the hips and legs. This is true for running, throwing, and jumping actions which may be the final performance objective or a component of more complex movements. For example, often the energy of motion generated in the hips and legs is transferred up through the midsection by bending, extending, twisting, or flexing, and finally is received by the upper body to execute some type of skilled movement involving shoulders, chest, and arms.

The organization of plyometric exercises in Part III follows the power-chain concept. The majority of exercises are specific to leg and hip action because these muscle groups are really the center of power of athletic movement and have major involvement in virtually all sports. Plyometric movements designed to work the musculature of

the hips and legs and the specific muscle actions affected are described below.

Bounds The emphasis in bounding is to gain maximum height as well as horizontal distance. Bounds are performed either with both feet together or in alternate fashion, as shown in the drawing below.

The functional anatomy of bounding involves flexion of the thigh by the

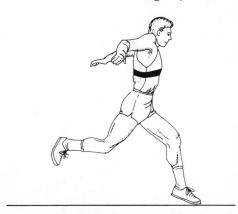

sartorius, iliacus, and gracilis; extension of the knee by the rectus femoris, vastus lateralis, medialis, and intermedius (quadraceps group); extension of the thigh by the biceps femoris, semitendinosus, and semimembranosus (hamstring group) and also by the gluteus maximus and minimus (the gluteals); flexion of the knee and foot by the gastrocnemius; adduction and abduction of the thigh by the gluteals and the adductor longus, brevis, magnus, minimus, and hallucis.

Hops The primary emphasis in hopping is to achieve maximum vertical height and a maximum rate of leg movement; gaining horizontal distance with the body is of secondary importance. Hops are performed either with both legs or one at a time.

The functional anatomy of hopping involves flexion of the thigh by the sartorius, iliacus, and gracilis; extension of the knee by the tensor fasciae latae, vastus lateralis, medialis, intermedius and rectus femoris; extension of the thigh and flexion of the leg by the biceps femoris, semitendinosus, and semimembranosus and also by the gluteus maximus and minimus; flexion of the knee and foot by the gastrocnemius, peroneus, and soleus; adduction and abduction of the thigh by the gluteus medius and minimus, and the adductor longus, brevis, magnus, minimus, and hallucis.

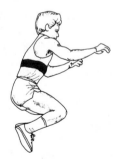

Jumps Attaining maximum height is sought in jumping, whereas rate of execution is secondary and horizontal distance is not even sought when jumping. Jumps can be performed

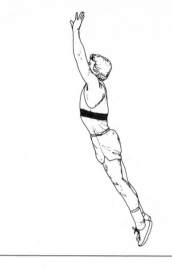

with both legs, one leg at a time, or in alternating fashion.

The functional anatomy of jumping involves flexion of the thigh by the sartorius, iliacus, and gracilis; extension of the knee by the vastus lateralis, medialis, intermedius, and the rectus femoris; extension of the thigh and flexion of the leg by the biceps femoris, semitendinosus, and semimembranosus and also by the gluteus maximus; adduction of the thigh by the gluteus medius and minimus and the adductor longus, brevis, magnus, minimus, and hallucis.

Leaps Leaping is a single-effort exercise in which both maximum height and horizontal distance are emphasized. Leaps are performed with either one or both legs.

The functional anatomy of leaping involves extension of the thigh by the

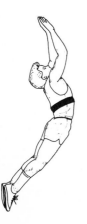

biceps femoris, semitendinosus, and semimembranosus, and by the gluteus maximus and minimus; extension of the knee by the vastus lateralis, medialis, and intermedius; flexion of the thigh and pelvis by the tensor fasciae latae, sartorius, iliacus, and gracilis; adduction and abduction of the thigh by the gluteus medius and minimus, and the adductor longus, brevis, and magnus.

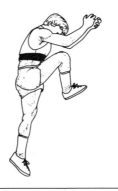

Skips Skipping is performed in an alternating hop-step manner that emphasizes both height and horizontal distance.

The functional anatomy of skipping involves extension of the thigh by the biceps femoris, semitendinosus, and semimembranosus, and by the gluteus minimus and maximus; flexion of the thigh by the tensor fasciae latae, sartorious, iliacus, and gracilis; extension of the foot by the gastrocnemius.

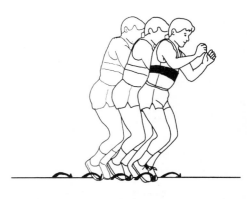

Ricochets The emphasis in ricocheting is solely on rapid rate of leg and foot movement; minimizing vertical and horizontal distance allows for a higher rate of execution.

The functional anatomy of ricocheting involves extension of the knee and hip joint by the vastus lateralis, medialis, and intermedius; flexion of the thigh by the sartorius, pectineus, adductor brevis, adductor longus, and tensor fasciae latae.

Landis (1983) describes the midsection or trunk as the body's shock absorber and likens it to the connecting link of the power chain between the "tractor" (hips and legs) and the "trailer" (upper body). An often neglected area of exercise, the trunk is extremely important in efficient and powerful execution of many athletic movements. Plyometric exercises designed specifically for the trunk are the following:

Swings These are movements of the trunk that are lateral, horizontal, or vertical, with secondary involvement of shoulders, chest, and arms.

The functional anatomy of swinging involves rotation of the spine and pelvis by the obliquus abdominus, transversus abdominus, serratus anterior and posterior; flexion and extension of the spine by the rectus

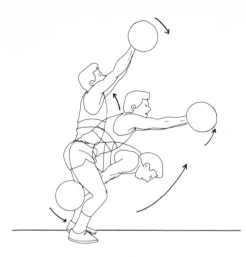

abdominus, transversus abdominus, obliquus externus, spinalis, longissimus thoracis, sacrospinalis, and semispinalis.

Twists Twisting is defined as the torquing and/or lateral movement of the torso without major involvement of the shoulders and arms.

The functional anatomy of twisting involves rotation of the spine and pelvis by the rectus abdominus, transversus abdominus, obliquus externus, and obliquus internus abdominus.

In many sports the end result of the power generated in the hips and legs and transferred through the midsection is seen as actions involving the chest, shoulders, back, and arms. Thus movements such as throwing, catching, pushing, pulling and swinging are primarily upper body activities; however, more careful analysis reveals that the trunk, hips, and legs also play important roles of support, weight transfer and balance. Thrusts, throws, strokes, passes, and swings all engage various muscle groups of the upper body. The relative degree of arm and shoulder movement differentiates these

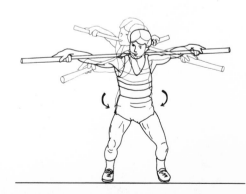

action sequences. The functional
anatomy of these movements is fairly
similar and involves integrated flexion,
extension, and abduction of the arms
by the pectoralis major and minor,
serratus anterior, triceps brachii,
brachialis, and biceps brachii; support
of the arms and shoulder girdle
throughout flexion and extension by
deltoideus, rhomboideus major and
minor, trapezius, coracobrachialis,
subclavius, and latissimus dorsi.

Chapter 4 EXECUTION GUIDELINES

In training with plyometric exercises, just as with other forms of athletic training, certain guidelines for proper and effective performance must be followed. Some of the guidelines have been mentioned in chapter 2; in this chapter other key aspects of plyometric training are emphasized.

Guideline 1
WARM UP/
WARM DOWN

Because plyometric exercises demand flexibility and agility, all drills should be preceded by an adequate period of warm-up and followed by a proper

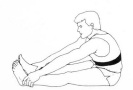

warm-down. Jogging, form running, stretching, and simple calisthenics are strongly recommended before and after every workout.

Guideline 2
HIGH INTENSITY

Intensity is an important factor in plyometric training. Quickness of exe-

cution with maximal effort is essential for optimal training effects. The rate of muscle stretch is more important than the magnitude of the stretch. A greater reflex response is achieved when the muscle is loaded rapidly. Because the exercises must be performed intensely, it is important to take adequate rest between successive exercise sequences.

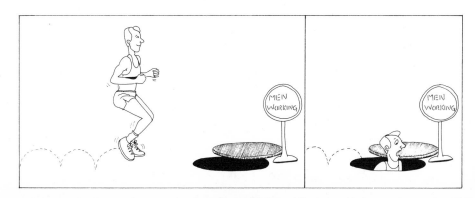

Guideline 3
PROGRESSIVE OVERLOAD

A plyometric training program must provide for resistive, temporal, and spatial overload. Overload forces the muscles to work at greater intensities. Proper overload is regulated by controlling the heights from which athletes drop, the weights used, and the distances covered. Improper overload may negate the effectiveness of the exercise or may even cause injury. Thus, using weights that exceed the resistive overload demands of certain plyometric movements may increase strength but not necessarily explosive power. Resistive overload in most plyometric exercises takes the form of forces of momentum and gravity, using objects relatively light in weight such as medicine balls or dumbbells, or merely body weight.

Guideline 4
MAXIMIZE FORCE/ MINIMIZE TIME

Both force and velocity of movement are important in plyometric training. In many cases the critical concern is the speed at which a particular action can be performed. For example, in shot-putting the primary objective is to exert maximum force throughout the putting movement. The quicker the action sequence is executed, the greater the force generated and the longer the distance achieved.

Guideline 5
PERFORM THE OPTIMAL NUMBER OF REPETITIONS

Usually the number of repetitions ranges from eight to 10, with fewer repetitions for more exerting sequences and more repetitions for those exer-

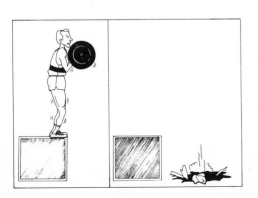

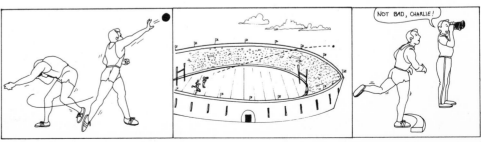

cises involving less overall effort. The number of sets also may vary accordingly. Various East German studies (Gambetta, 1981) suggest six to 10 sets for most exercises, while the Russian literature (Veroshanski, 1966) recommends from three to six sets especially for some of the more intense jumping drills.

It is important to understand that most plyometric drills fall into one of two categories: single-response (SR) or multiple-response (MR) drills. The former represent a single, intense effort such as employed in take-offs, initial bursts of motion, and releases. The latter are also intense but they place more emphasis on stamina and overall speed by involving several efforts in succession. Actually, the same drill can be worked either way. For example, the Depth Jump described in chapter 5 is basically a single drop from a box, followed by a high vertical jump. Yet by placing a row of cones in front of the box and doing a series of jumps over them, the athlete is performing a multiple-response drill (see below). A good plyometric program utilizes both types of responses, thus working both the more specific and the overall action efforts.

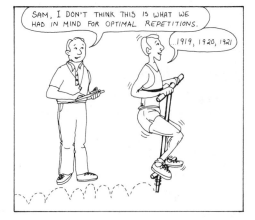

Sometimes the number of repetitions is dictated not only by intensity of the drill but also by the athlete's condition, the execution of each repetition, and the value of the outcome. Remember that these drills are being performed to improve nerve-muscle reactions, explosiveness, quickness, and the ability to generate forces in certain directions. An athlete will only benefit from the number of repetitions done well. For example, if he or she performs a set of hops, bounds, or throws correctly for eight repetitions but begins to fatigue and performs incorrectly thereafter, then eight repetitions is enough. In plyometrics training little is gained with low intensity, poorly executed exercises.

The number of sets, repetitions, and rest periods recommended in Part III are based on our experiences of teaching and coaching plyometric training at the junior high, high school, professional, and elite athlete levels, and on research literature for particular drills. They are not absolutes, but merely a basis from which you can begin. Adjust these values within the objectives outlined here to achieve your optimal training objectives.

Guideline 6
REST PROPERLY

A rest period of 1 to 2 minutes between sets is usually sufficient for the neuromuscular systems stressed by plyometric exercises to recuperate. An adequate period of rest between plyometric training days also is important for proper recovery of muscles, ligaments, and tendons. Two to 3 days per week of plyometric training seems to give optimal results. It is important not to precede plyometrics, especially jump drills and other leg movements, with heavy weight workouts of the lower body. Previously fatigued muscles, tendons, and ligaments can become overstressed by the high resistive loads placed on them during the plyometric workout.

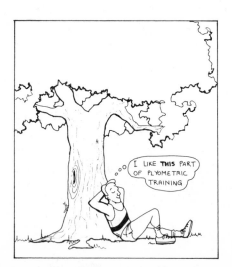

Guideline 7
BUILD A PROPER FOUNDATION FIRST

Because a strength base is advantageous in plyometrics, a weight training program should be designed to complement, not retard, development of explosive power.

Establishing a strength base prior to plyometric training need not be overdone. Veroshanski and Chernousov (1974) suggest a maximum squat of two times body weight before attempting depth jumps and similar plyometrics. This is an extreme criterion

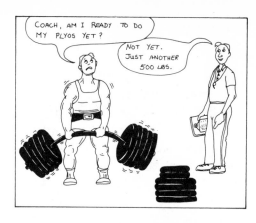

and one that we feel is unnecessary for successful performance and positive training effect using plyometrics. Other researchers (Valik, 1966) corroborate our contention in their application of plyometric training in 12- to 14-year-olds as preparation for future strength training. And this is also supported by McFarlane (1982), who suggests moderate jump training with 14-year-olds and older youths. Sinclair (1981) notes there does not appear to be any significant response to explosive strength training in the adolescent until after the onset of puberty; therefore training programs should be prescribed with care.

Beginners should start with moderate drills such as jumps from ground level, and hops, bounds, and leaps with both legs. As strength and explosive power increase, a progression to one-legged drills, depth jumps and decline and incline work can be initiated. Strength and flexibility training of abdominal muscles and lower back muscles are recommended for several weeks prior to doing skips, swings, and similar trunk exercises.

Guideline 8
INDIVIDUALIZE THE TRAINING PROGRAM

For best results, you will want to individualize the plyometric training program, which means you should know what each athlete is capable of doing and just how much training is beneficial. Unfortunately, little research has been aimed at testing a person's capabilities and determining how much training is optimal. As with so many other areas of sports training, individualizing the plyometric training program is more of an art than a science.

The intensity and amount of overload are two critical variables here. Because the research is so scarce, views differ as to the optimum intensity and overload for different plyometric exercises. Coaches from Eastern Bloc countries recommend that athletes be able to barbell squat 1.5 to 2 times their body weight in order to train with certain plyometric exercises, but this criterion is not based on research evidence and does not apply to all plyometric exercises, nor is it appropriate for every individual. Thus, many leaders in the field are calling for simple tests to provide some basis for individualizing the training, even if these tests are not based on a substantial body of research evidence.

A notable exception to the absence of research concerns the depth jump exercise. Bosco and Komi (1979, 1981) and Veroshanski (1967) have examined the optimal height for executing depth jumps. Their results indicate that dropping from a height of 29 inches develops speed, whereas dropping from 43 inches develops dynamic strength more. Above 43 inches, the time and energy it takes to cushion the force of the drop to the ground defeats the purpose for plyometric training.

Based on the work of Sinclair (1981) and Costello (1984), as well as on our own work in guiding the plyometric training of many athletes, we have identified four basic tests we believe are helpful in evaluating power. The testing procedures for these tests are given in Appendix B:

1. Vertical jump;
2. Depth jump heights;
3. Box jump tests;
4. Medicine ball pass.

At this time we cannot give you norms for interpreting test scores and individualizing the training program.

Instead, we suggest you give these four tests before beginning plyometric exercise training, then retest approximately every third week of the program. If you do not see any improvement, try to evaluate whether the intensity of the training and the overload is too little or too much. If you are a coach, ask for the athlete's opinion about the training; then use good judgment in adjusting the intensity and overload of the workout.

By systematically monitoring the progress and testing for change, you will have a better basis for making adjustments in training. Perhaps if you will keep records, and if others will do the same, collectively we will have a basis for developing norms from the tests—and thus better prescriptions for training.

OTHER EXECUTION GUIDELINES

As mentioned in chapter 2, specificity training in plyometrics is important

as strength and endurance training. Generally, plyometric exercises should be performed at amplitudes and intensities corresponding closely to the power movements and action sequences of specific sport skills. In some cases, however, purposeful temporal and spatial exaggerations are recommended as overload mechanisms.

Research by Bosco and Komi (1979) shows that the performance of jumps with undamped (without delay) landings result in higher power and force values than those with damped (added flexion) landings. The difference between these two types of landings is illustrated above, right. Thus, the quicker the person switches from yielding work to overcoming work, the more powerful the response. In most cases, a good guideline to follow is that athletes should execute undamped landings in jumping exercises.

Proper foot placement when doing the yielding and overcoming work is essential. In order to obtain as quick a release as possible, the athlete must

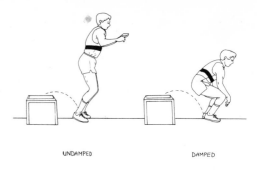

UNDAMPED   DAMPED

maintain a locked ankle when landing on the ground. Rolling the foot from heel to toe (see below) or allowing movement along the ankle joint slows down the response and displaces the force away from the overcoming portion. The best way to land on the

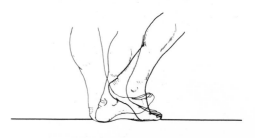

WRONG

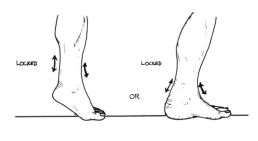

LOCKED OR LOCKED

RIGHT

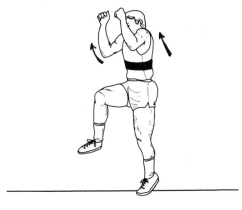

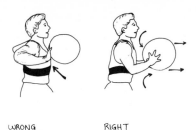

WRONG   RIGHT

thumbs-up position helps to counteract this tendency by forcing the torso to remain in a more upright position, thus aiding balance.

ground is on the ball of the foot, although this is easier said than done. A flat-footed landing is okay, but with practice the former method can be learned and should always be remembered for obtaining maximum benefits from lower limb plyometric drills.

In all plyometric jumps, hops, leaps, bounds, skips, and ricochets, concentrate on "knees-up/thumbs-up." This helps in keeping balance, centering the workload around the hips and legs, and developing additional power movements with the upper body. When knees are brought upward abruptly, the tendency is for the shoulders to drop forward. Holding the hands in the

Follow-through is important in plyometric movements involving upper body muscle groups. Force should be applied continuously and quickness of action should be emphasized. In repetitive thrusts and throws, such as the medicine ball throw (see top right) or the heavy bag thrust, try to prevent the recovery or "catch" phase from go-

ing beyond the point of full extension or flexion. This will ensure that limb and trunk musculature is properly stretched (loaded) so as to initiate a more forceful, reactive explosion.

This concludes our list of guidelines for executing the plyometric drills presented in the next part. We suggest you reread this chapter after having practiced plyometric drills several times to help you become more aware of the execution guidelines.

Part III PLYOMETRIC DRILLS

There is probably no limit to the variety of plyometric exercises that can be devised. Some imagination and inquisitiveness, peppered with a basic understanding of neuromuscular processes involved, allow for the development of useful plyometric drills. However, it is neither practical nor necessary to analyze each movement pattern of every sport skill and design a plyometric drill for that specific skill. In fact, there are a relatively small number of key power movements in sport, and a set of drills for these power movements is presented here in Part III. Coaches and athletes will see quite readily which of these plyometric drills are more appropriate for their own training needs; our explanations and demonstrations are intended to add a few insights.

The exercises begin with the simpler, more fundamental drills and progress to the more complex and difficult. As the athlete improves in strength and agility, and in exercise performance, then he or she can advance to the more difficult drills.

We would like to add a word of caution here: Although plyometric exercises done properly and under appropriate supervision offer no greater risk than other exercise programs or sports participation, carelessness in bounding, jumping, leaping, hopping, and so on can result in injury. Coaches, and athletes as well, should judge whether athletes have the motor skills for properly executing the more complex drills that involve stair climbing or changing directions using the various apparatus illustrated here in Part III. Also, in order to avoid fatigue and reduce risk of injury, no more than three or four drills should be performed in a workout.

Do not let plyometrics deprive you of sport participation through injury. Instead, let the proper and safe execution of plyometrics enhance your sport performance.

Chapter 5 LEGS AND HIPS

BOUNDS

Drill: Double Leg Bound

This exercise develops explosive power in the muscles of the legs and hips, specifically the gluteals, hamstrings, quadriceps, and gastrocnemius. Arm and shoulder muscles also are indirectly involved. The drill has wide application to a number of different sports including jumping, running, weightlifting, and competitive swimming.

Starting position

Begin the exercise from a half-squat stance. Arms should be down at the sides, with shoulders forward and out over the knees. Keep the back straight and hold the head up.

Action sequence

Jump outward and upward, using the extension of the hips and forward

thrusting movement of the arms. Try to attain maximum height and distance by fully straightening the body. Upon landing, resume the starting

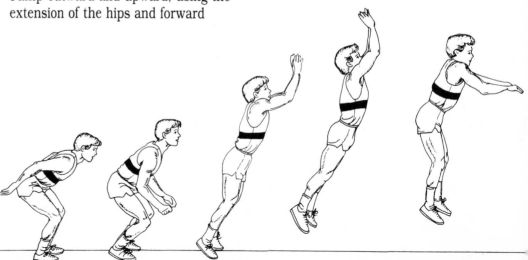

position and initiate the next bound. Emphasize "reaching for the sky."

Perform 3 to 5 sets of 8 to 12 repetitions with about 2 minutes rest between each set.

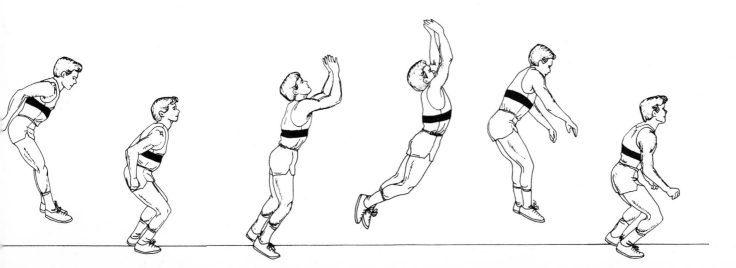

Drill: Alternate Leg Bound

This drill is very similar to the double leg bound in developing explosive leg and hip power. Alternating the legs specifically works the flexors and extensors of the thighs and hips, a drill that is used to enhance running, striding, and sprinting actions.

Starting position

Assume a comfortable stance with one foot slightly ahead of the other as to initiate a step; arms should be relaxed and at the sides.

Action sequence

Begin by pushing off with the back leg, driving the knee up to the chest and attempting to gain as much height and distance as possible before landing. Quickly extend outward with the driving foot. Either swing the arms in a contralateral motion or execute a double arm swing. Repeat the sequence (driving with the other leg) upon landing. A variation of this is to begin the sequence with a 10-yard run proceeding immediately into the bounds.

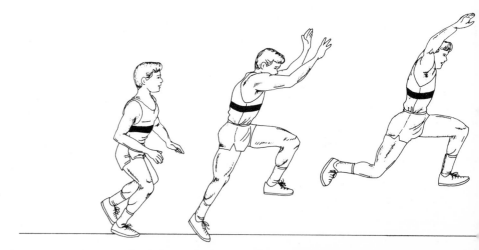

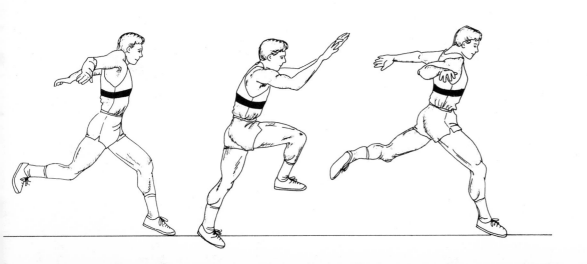

Drill: Double Leg Box Bound

This drill requires 2 to 4 boxes ranging from about 12 to 22 inches in height. Use of the boxes places greater overloads on the same muscle groups engaged in the double leg bound. This exercise requires more stability of the lower back and trunk areas. (See Appendix C for building the boxes required for this drill.)

Starting position

With the boxes spaced evenly 3 to 6 feet apart, stand approximately 2 to 3 steps in front of the first box. Feet should be slightly more than shoulder-width apart. The body is held in a semi-squat stance with back straight, head up, and arms at the sides.

Action sequence

As in double leg bounds, begin by exploding upward onto the first box; as soon as you land on the box, explode upward again as high and as far out as possible, landing on the ground.

Repeat this sequence using the second box and the third, and so on, until completed.

Perform 4 to 6 sets using 2 to 4 boxes, with about 2 minutes rest between each set.

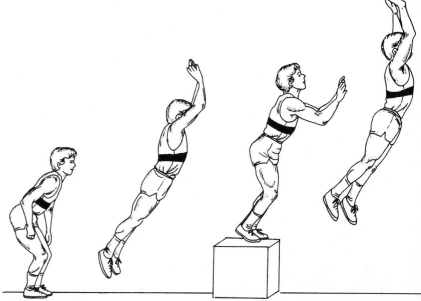

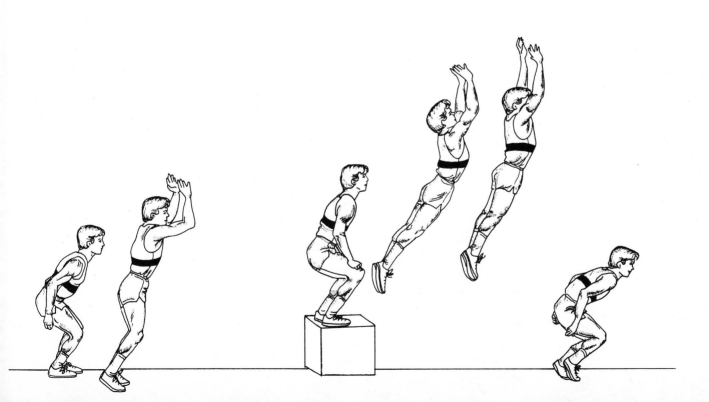

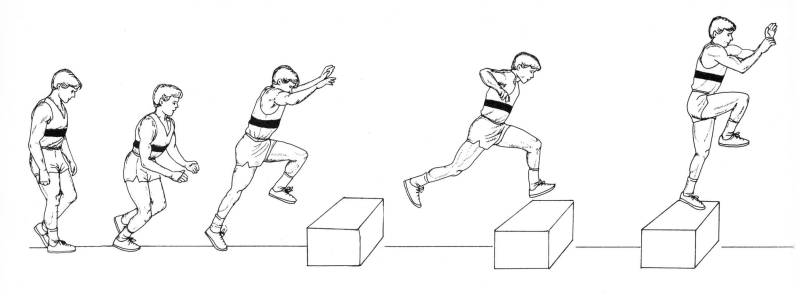

Drill:
Alternate Leg Box Bound

By incorporating the use of 2 to 4 boxes (approximately 12 to 22 inches in height), this drill places overloads on the leg flexors and hip extensors by alternately bounding on each leg.

Starting position
Assume the same stance as in the alternate leg bound, 2 to 3 steps in front of a series of boxes spaced approximately 3 to 6 feet apart.

Action sequence
The action sequence for this exercise is the same as that described for the alternate leg bound except that every other step is made from a box.

Perform 5 to 8 sets of 2 to 4 boxes, with 2 minutes rest between each set.

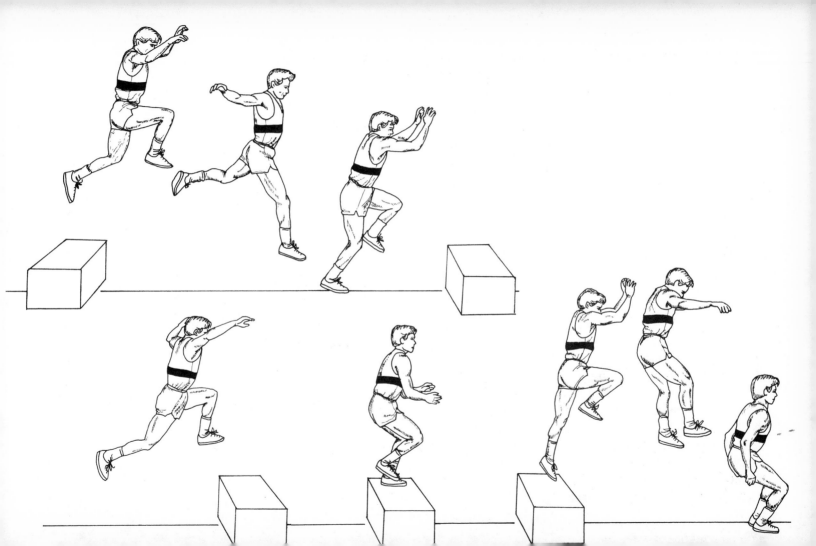

Drill: Incline Bound

This drill is performed on a sloped hill (about 20 degrees inclination), stairs, or stadium steps. By working uphill, a constant resistive force or overload is placed on the muscle systems used for bounding. This constant overload helps to develop strength and power. Both double and alternate leg variations of the incline bound are suggested.

Starting position

Assume the same stance as in the double leg bound at the bottom of the hill or steps.

Action sequence

Performance is similar to double and alternate leg bounds. Begin by exploding upward from step to step gradually increasing the number of steps or distance as skill and power improve. Use the arms in an upward thrusting motion to help achieve a high lifting action. When performing double leg incline bounds, keep the feet about shoulder-width apart. In alternate leg incline bounds, stride with each foot as far as possible. The arm action can be contralateral or a double-arm pump.

Perform 4 to 6 sets of 10 to 20 bounds with about 2 minutes rest between each set.

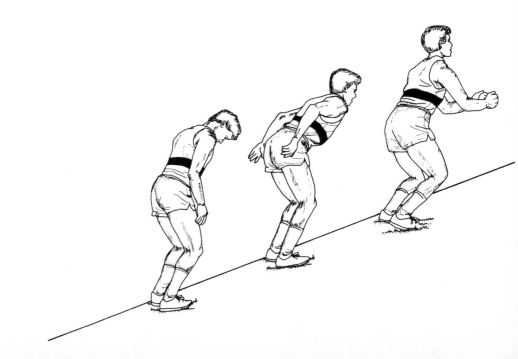

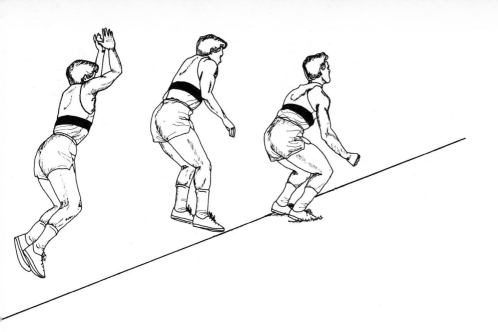

Drill: Lateral Bound

This drill requires angle boxes, a grassy hill, or similar incline, but regular boxes can be substituted if angle boxes are not available. This exercise emphasizes use of the thigh adductor and abductor muscles as well as those in the hips, thighs, and lower back. The stabilizer muscles of the knee and ankle are also used. The lateral bound is excellent for skating, hockey, Nordic skiing, tennis, basketball, and baseball.

Starting position
Assume a semi-squat stance at the side of the angle box or incline approximately 1 long step away.

Action sequence
Push off with the outside foot moving laterally onto the box, and concentrate on obtaining height and lateral distance. Upon landing, drive off again in the opposite direction, attempting to gain as much lateral distance as possible.

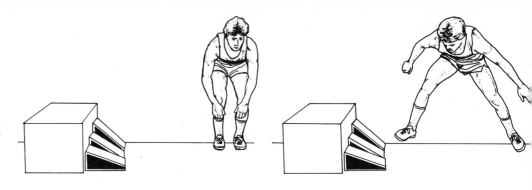

Perform 3 to 6 sets of 8 to 12 repetitions; a rest period of 1 to 2 minutes is adequate between sets.

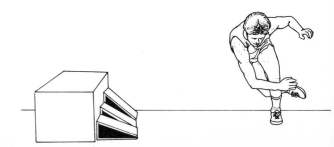

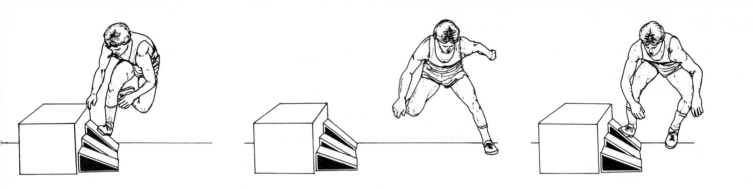

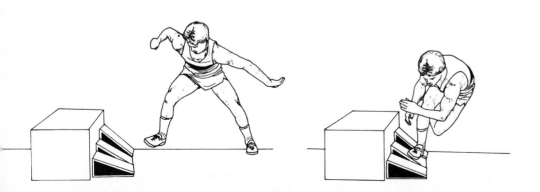

HOPS

Drill: Double Leg Speed Hop

This exercise develops speed and power in the muscles of the legs and hips, specifically working the gluteals, hamstrings, quadriceps, and gastrocnemius at a rapid and powerful rate. It is a useful exercise for developing the speed and explosiveness required when running.

Starting position

Assume a relaxed upright stance with back straight, head up, and shoulders slightly forward. Keep arms at sides and bent at 90 degrees with the thumbs up.

Action sequence

Begin by jumping upward as high as possible, flexing the legs completely so as to bring the feet under the buttocks. Emphasize maximum lift by bringing the knees high and forward with each repetition. Upon each landing, jump quickly upward again with the same cycling action of the legs, using the arms to help achieve maximum lift.

The action sequence should be executed as rapidly as possible. Work at gaining height and distance, but not at the expense of repetition rate.

Perform 3 to 6 sets of 10 to 20 repetitions, with 1 to 2 minutes rest between each set.

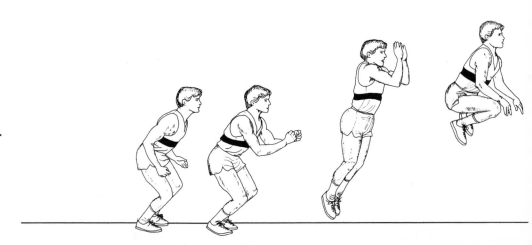

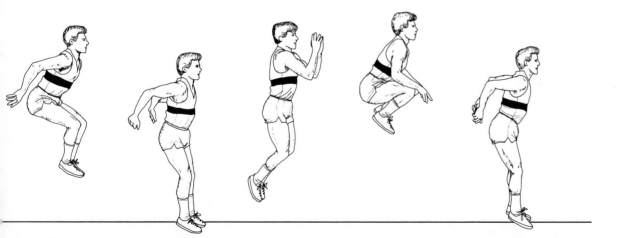

Drill: Single Leg Speed Hop

This drill is similar to the double leg speed hop except that it is done with one leg. This places an overload on the muscles of the hips, legs, and lower back; it also incorporates the muscles that stabilize the knee and ankle.

Starting position

Assume the same stance as in the double leg speed hop except that one leg should be held in a stationary flexed position throughout the exercise.

Action sequence

Begin the exercise as in the double leg hop but with one (the same) leg at a time.

Perform 2 to 4 sets of 8 to 12 repetitions on each leg, with approximately 2 minutes rest between each set.

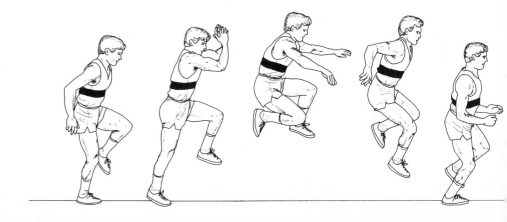

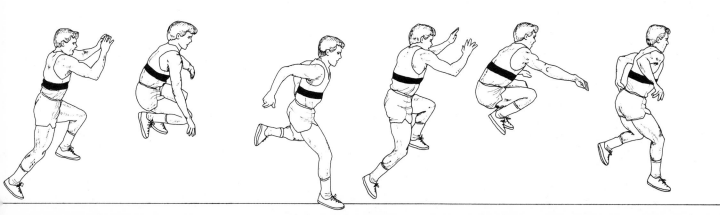

Drill:
Incremental Vertical Hop

For this exercise you will need a rope or rubber surgical tubing approximately 15 feet in length. Attach one end to a wall or pole at a height of about 4 feet and the other end to a cone, tire, or similar movable object at ground level. This is excellent for basketball, volleyball, and track and field activities.

Starting position

Assume a relaxed position immediately to the side of the lowest end of the rope with feet together, facing the wall or pole. The arms should be cocked, ready to aid in providing lift.

Action sequence

Hopping back and forth over the rope, try to advance toward the wall (up the rope) as high as possible. Bring the knees forward and upward toward the chest while tucking the feet underneath the buttocks. Continue up the rope as far as possible, thus completing the set.

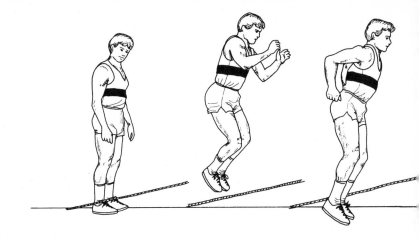

Perform 3 to 6 sets of as many repetitions as possible. Rest periods of 1 to 2 minutes between each set are recommended.

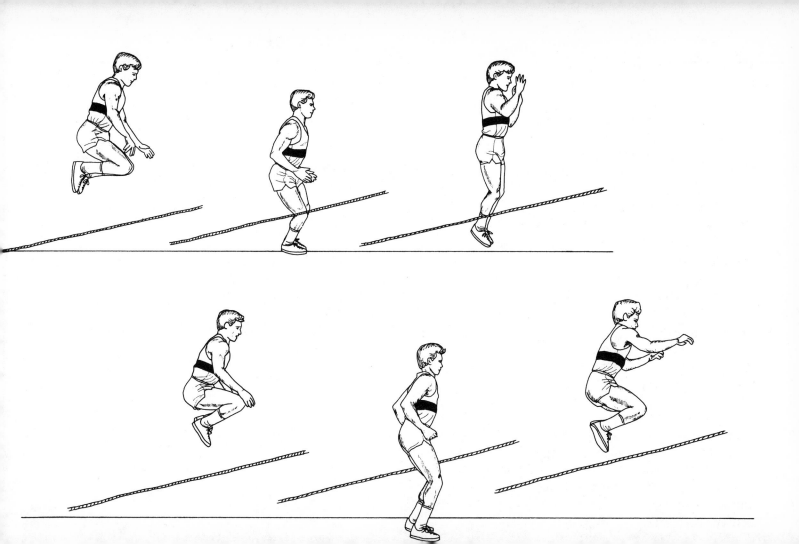

Drill: Decline Hop

Use a grassy hill of about 2 to 4 degrees inclination. (*Note:* Do not attempt this exercise on steps, bleachers, or a wet, slick surface.) This drill develops speed and strength of the legs and hips, specifically the quadriceps, hamstrings, gluteals, and lower back, through increased shock on the musculature and increased speed due to the downward momentum.

Starting position

Assume a quarter-squat stance at the top of the hill with the body facing down the fall line.

Action sequence

Execution of this movement is the same as that described for the double leg hop. However, performing this hop on the decline requires even greater emphasis on repetition rate and speed of movement. The single leg decline hop is suggested only after mastering the double leg hop.

Do 4 to 6 sets of 6 to 10 repetitions, with approximately 2 minutes rest between each set.

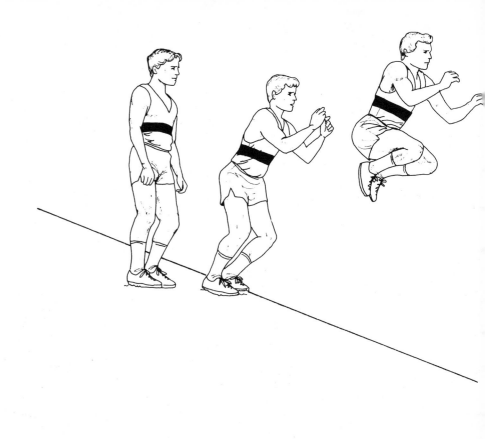

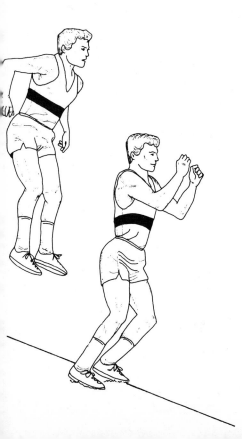

Drill: Side Hop

This exercise involves the use of 2 cones approximately 18 to 26 inches in height. The movement specifically develops the thigh abductor muscles, stabilizers of the knees and ankles, and enhances explosive lateral power throughout the legs and hips. This drill is very useful for all activities employing lateral movement.

Starting position

Set both cones side by side approximately 2 to 3 feet apart. Assume a relaxed upright stance to the outside of one of the cones. The feet should be together and pointing straight ahead, and the arms cocked ready to provide lift and aid in balance.

Action sequence

From the starting position, jump sideways over the first cone and then the second one. Without hesitating, change direction by jumping back over the second cone and then the first one; continue this back-and-forth sequence. Use the arms in an upward thrusting motion with thumbs up and elbows at 90 degrees.

Perform 5 to 8 sets of 6 to 12 repetitions, with 1 to 2 minutes rest between each set.

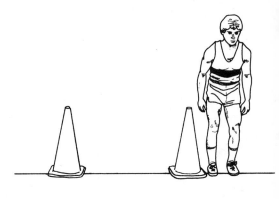

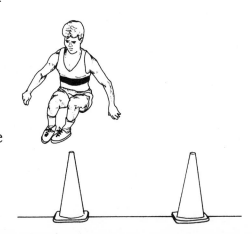

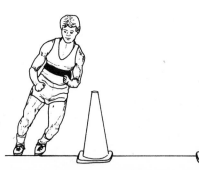

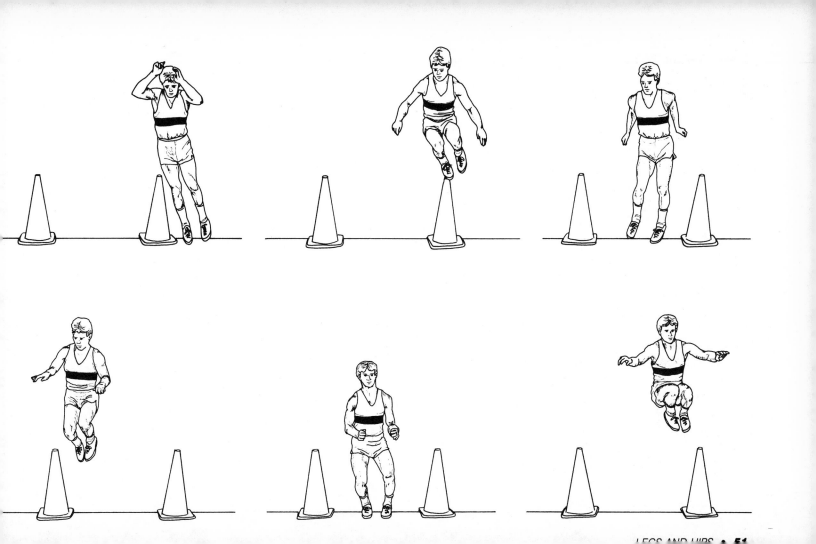

Drill: Angle Hop

This drill preferably is done on a multiple angle box or similar apparatus, which must be securely attached to the ground so as not to move or slip while the hops are being performed. The angle hop develops explosive power and speed of reaction in the thigh adductors and ankle stabilizers, and improves balance and lateral movement. This drill is useful in Alpine skiing, tennis, football, and gymnastics, as well as other sports.

Starting position
Stand in a relaxed position on one of the angled surfaces of the box.

Action sequence
Hop laterally from one side of the box to the next sequentially, emphasizing a rapid side-to-side motion. Once skill has improved, progress to more distant angles. Hold the arms out and up to aid in balance.

Perform 4 to 8 sets of 8 to 12 repetitions with about 2 minutes rest between each set.

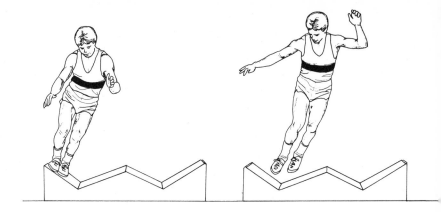

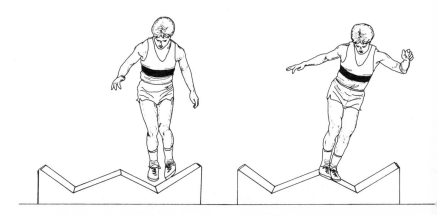

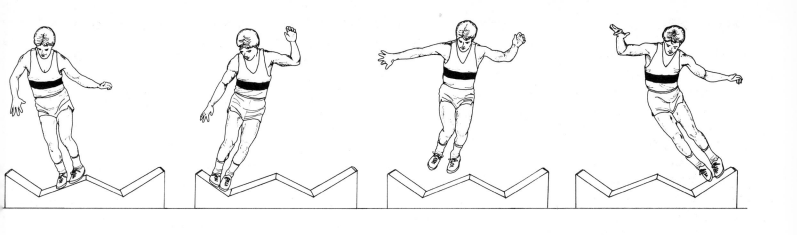
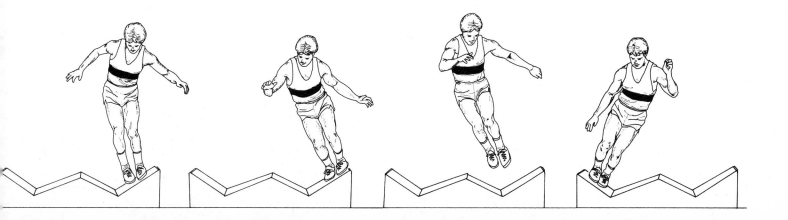

JUMPS

Drill: Squat Jump

This exercise is performed on a flat semi-resilient surface. It is a basic drill for developing power in the hip flexors, quadriceps, gastrocnemius, hamstrings, and gluteals and is applicable to many sports. The primary emphasis in the squat jump is to attain maximum height with every effort.

Starting position

Assume a relaxed upright stance with feet placed about shoulder-width apart. Interlock the fingers and place the palms of the hands against the back of the head. This will minimize involvement of the arms, thus emphasizing involvement of the legs and hips.

Action sequence

Begin by quickly dropping downward to a half-squat position; immediately check this downward movement and explode upward as high as possible. Upon landing, repeat the sequence; on each repetition, initiate the jumping phase just prior to reaching the half-

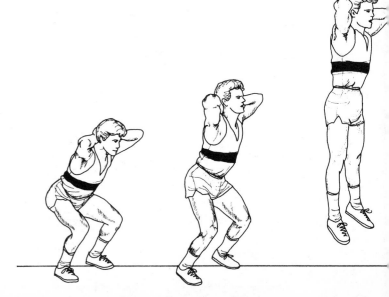

squat starting position. Work for maximum height with each jump.

Two to 4 sets of 15 to 30 repetitions are suggested; rest 2 minutes between sets.

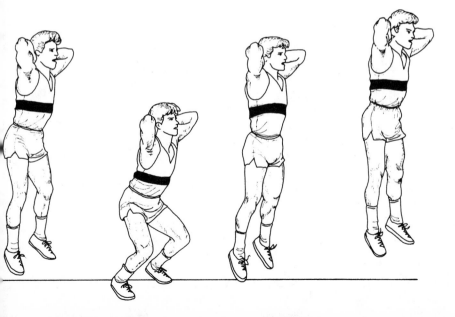

Drill: Knee-Tuck Jump

Knee-tuck jumps are done on a resilient, flat surface such as grass or a wrestling mat. This drill is performed as a series of rapid explosive jumps that exercise the hip and leg flexors, gastrocnemius, gluteals, quadriceps, and hamstrings.

Starting position

Assume a comfortable upright stance, placing the hands palms down at chest height.

Action sequence

Begin by rapidly dipping down to about the quarter-squat level and immediately explode upward. Drive the knees high toward the chest and attempt to touch them to the palms of the hands. Upon landing, repeat the sequence, each time thinking of driving the knees upward and tucking the feet under the body. Repetitions are performed at a fairly rapid rate with minimum contact on the ground.

Two to 4 sets of 10 to 20 repetitions with about 2 minutes rest between sets are recommended.

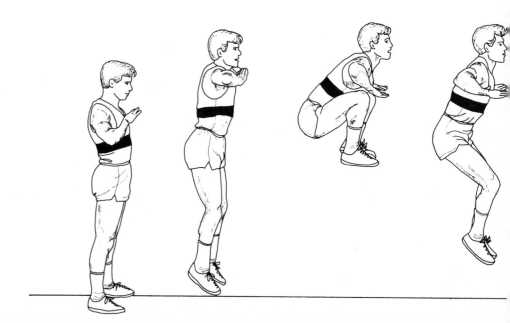

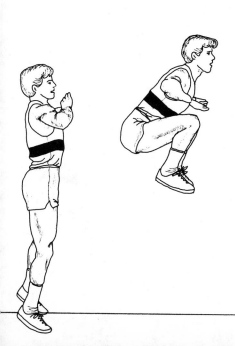

Drill: Split Jump

Split jumps are performed on a flat surface and affect the muscles of the lower back, hamstrings, gluteals, quadriceps, extensors, and flexors of the lower leg. Split jumps are especially good for developing striding power for running and cross-country skiing; they are also specific to the "split" portion of the clean and jerk.

Starting position

Assume a stance with one leg extended forward and the other oriented somewhat behind the midline of the body as in executing a long step or stride. The forward leg is flexed with a 90-degree bend at the knee.

Action sequence

Jump as high and straight up as possible. Use the arms in an upward swinging motion to gain additional lift. Upon landing, retain the spread-legged position, bending the knee of the forward leg to absorb the shock. After regaining stability, repeat the motion for the required number of times, going as high as possible each time. Upon completing the sequence (and rest), perform the exercise again with the opposite leg forward.

Perform 2 to 3 sets of 5 to 8 jumps with each extended leg. A rest period of about 1 to 2 minutes between sets is recommended.

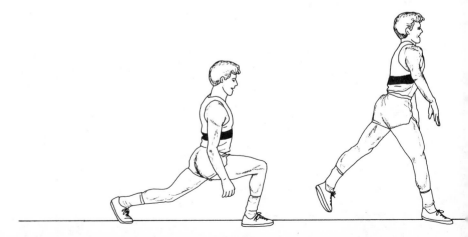

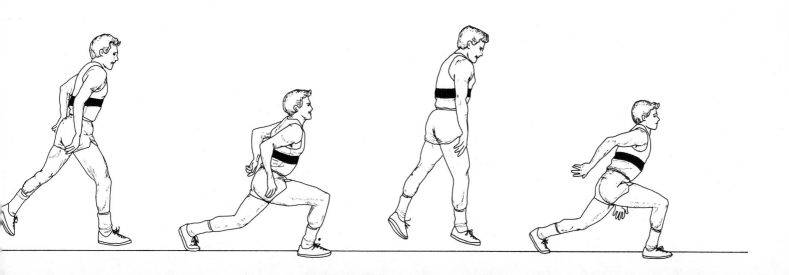

Drill: Scissor Jump

As in the split jump, this exercise works the muscles of the lower back, hip extensors, hamstrings, and quadriceps. It is very similar to the split jump except that leg speed also is emphasized; therefore, it is especially good for runners and jumpers.

Starting position

The beginning stance of the scissor jump is the same as that of the split jump.

Action sequence

The initial movement of the scissor jump also is identical to that of the split jump. However, at the apex of the jump the position of the legs is reversed, that is, front to back and back to front. The switching of the legs occurs in midair and must be done very quickly before landing. After landing, the jump is repeated, again reversing the position of the legs. Attainment of maximal vertical height and leg speed are stressed in this exercise. A variation of this exercise for the more advanced is the double scissor jump in which a complete cycle of the legs (i.e., front to back, back to front, and vice versa) is attempted while in the air, landing with the legs in their original position.

Two to 3 sets of 5 to 8 repetitions with about 2 minutes rest between each set are suggested.

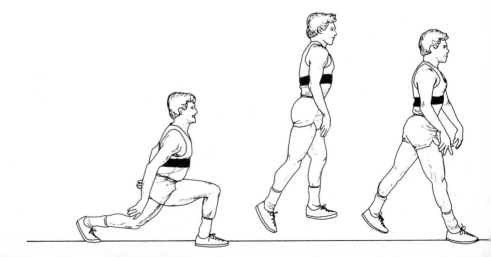

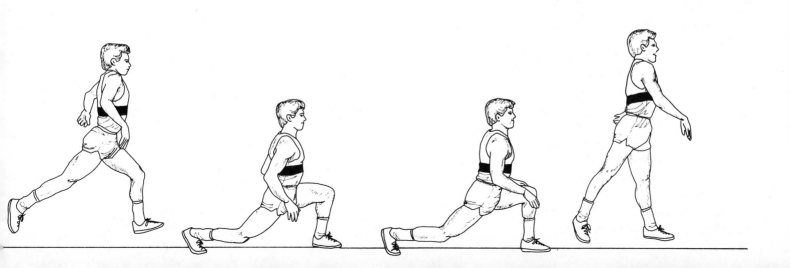

Drill: Box Jump

For this exercise you will need boxes, benches, or an elevated platform between 12 and 24 inches in height.

Starting position

Assume a relaxed stance facing the box or platform at a distance of about 18 to 20 inches away. Arms should be down at the sides and legs slightly bent.

Action sequence

Using the arms to aid in the initial burst, jump upward and forward, landing with feet together on top of the box or platform. Immediately jump back down to the original starting place and then repeat the sequence. A variation of this basic movement can be performed by alternating the directions of jumping onto and off the elevated surface. Remember to keep thumbs and knees up for balance and concentrate on rapidity of movement, minimizing contact time with ground and box.

Perform 3 to 6 sets of 8 to 12 jumps, with about 2 minutes rest between each set.

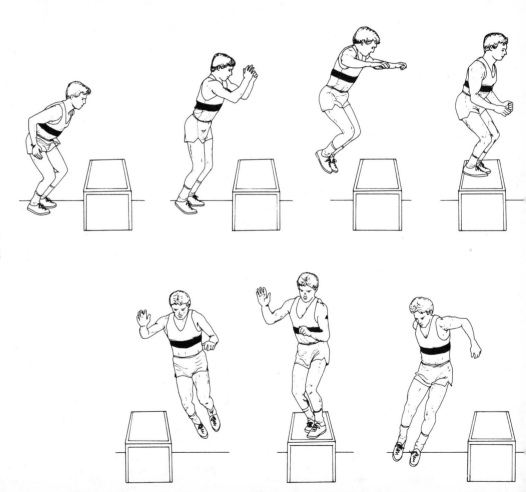

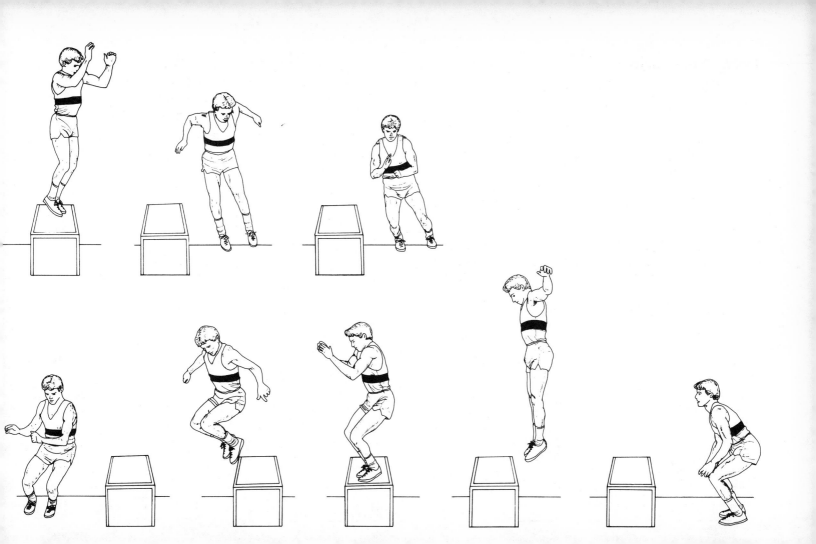

Drill: Depth Jump

An elevated surface (box or bench) approximately 25 to 45 inches in height is needed for this exercise. The landing surface should be fairly soft, such as grass or a wrestling mat. This is an especially good exercise for the quadriceps and hip girdle, as well as for the lower back and hamstrings. The depth jump is applicable to all sports because it employs leg strength, speed, and quickness.

Starting position

Begin by standing at the edge of the elevated platform with the front of the feet just over the edge. Keep the knees slightly bent and arms relaxed at the sides.

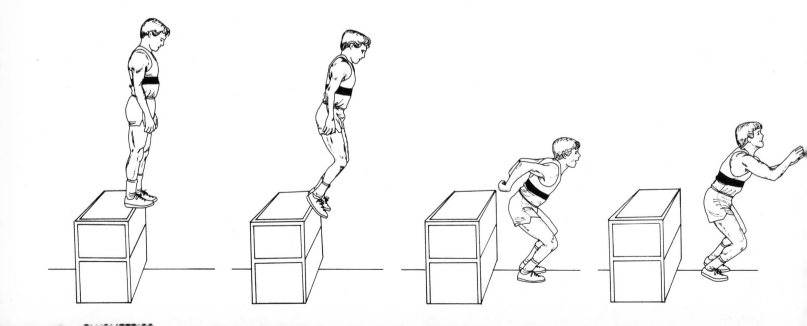

Action sequence

Drop from the elevated surface to the ground; do not jump off the platform. Land with both feet together and knees bent to absorb the shock of the landing phase. As soon as you land on the ground, initiate the jumping phase by swinging the arms upward and extending the body as high and as far out as possible. Maximum intensity and effort are required to gain optimal benefits. A variation is to perform an additional jump or two after the initial one. Keep knees and thumbs up for balance.

Do 3 to 6 sets of jumps, resting about 1 minute between each jump.

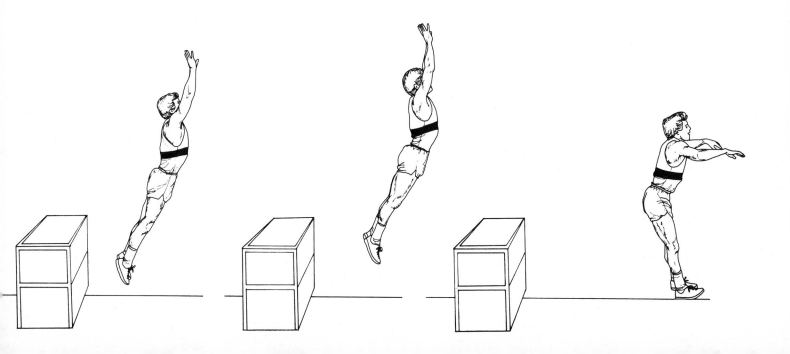

Drill:
Single Leg Stride Jump

A long sturdy bench, rectangular box, or a row of bleachers or stadium stairs is required for performing the stride jump, which involves the muscles of the lower back, quadriceps, gluteals, hamstrings, and hip flexors. This drill is excellent for cycling, football, basketball, and track and field jumping events.

Starting position

Assume a position to the side and at one end of the bench. Place the inside foot on top of the bench, with arms held downward at the sides.

Action sequence

Begin the exercise with an upward movement of the arms; then, using the inside leg (foot on bench) for power, jump upward as high as possible. Moving slightly forward down the bench, repeat the action as soon as the outside leg (away from the bench) touches the ground. Use mainly the inside leg for power and support, allowing the outside leg to barely touch the ground

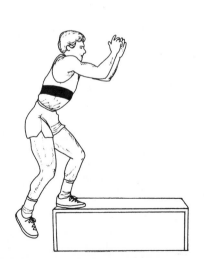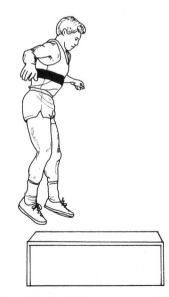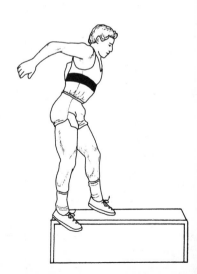

before jumping up again. Once the end of the bench is reached, turn around, and with leg positions reversed, repeat the sequence in the other direction. Remember to gain full height and body extension with each jump.

A workout of 2 to 4 sets of 6 to 10 repetitions with about 2 minutes rest between sets is suggested.

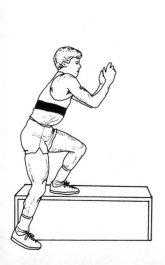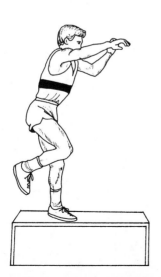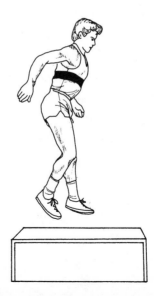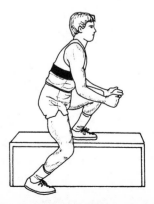

Drill:
Stride Jump Crossover

For this drill, the same type of equipment described in the single leg stride jump is needed. Quadriceps, gluteals, hamstrings, lower back muscles, gastrocnemius, and (indirectly) the shoulder girdle are all involved in this movement. The drill is useful for skills in basketball, football, cycling, gymnastics, and track and field jumping events.

Starting position

As in the single leg stride jump, assume a standing position at one end of the bench with one foot on the ground and the other on the bench. Arms should be down at the sides.

Action sequence

The movement is initiated by rapidly swinging the arms upward. This upward momentum is then continued by driving off the bench with the elevated leg, jumping as high as possible and extending the body fully. At this point

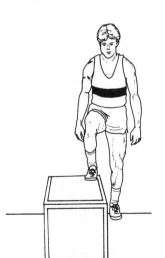
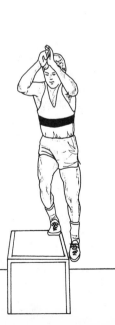
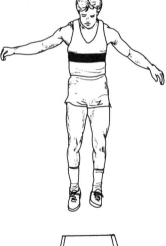
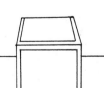
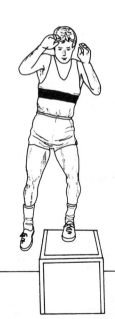

the body is carried over the bench and slightly forward so that the driving leg touches the ground on the opposite side of the bench and the trailing leg comes to rest on top of the bench. Orientation of the body and position of the feet are now just the opposite of the original starting position. As soon as the original driving leg makes contact with the ground, the motion is repeated but with the original trailing leg acting as the major power source. These movements are repeated back and forth the length of the bench. Work to achieve maximum height with each jump, using the arms to assist in lifting the body. Minimize ground and bench contact time with the feet; perform the movements as quickly and explosively as possible.

Two to 4 sets of 8 to 12 repetitions (with each driving leg) with a rest of about 1 to 2 minutes between each set are recommended.

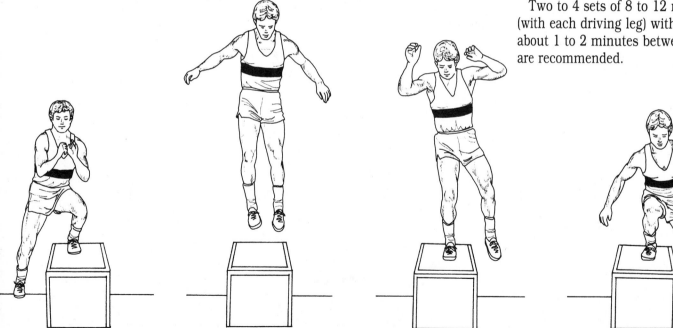

Drill: Side Jump/Sprint

A low bench, tackling dummy, or similar object for jumping over and cones for use as a finish line are required for this drill. This is a combination exercise going from a series of lateral jumps to a full sprint over a given distance. It involves the quadriceps, hamstrings, hip flexors, gastrocnemius, and gluteals and also practices the coordination required for rapid change of direction. This drill is applicable to tennis, basketball, baseball, football, and many other sports utilizing change of direction.

Starting position

Stand on one side of the bench with feet together and pointing straight ahead. Cones are placed 15 to 20 yards in front of the starting point to act as a finish line.

Action sequence

Begin by jumping back and forth over the bench for a designated number of repetitions (4 to 10). Upon landing on the last jump, go forward at a full sprint past the finish line. Two participants can do this exercise at the same time, using different benches or jumping objects. Obviously, the participant

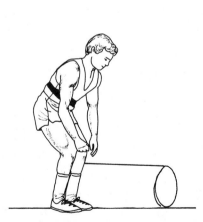
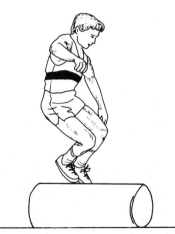
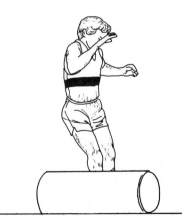

completing the designated number of jumps first will have an advantage in crossing the finish line first. This forces both participants to execute the side jumps as rapidly as possible, a primary objective of the drill. Anticipate the last landing and be ready to sprint forward. Emphasis is not on the height of the jumps but on the rate of execution. Keep the trunk and hips centered over the bench and carry the legs fluidly from side to side.

Perform the drill in 3 to 5 sets of 4 to 10 jumps and 1 sprint. Allow 1 to 2 minutes for recovery between jump/sprint sets.

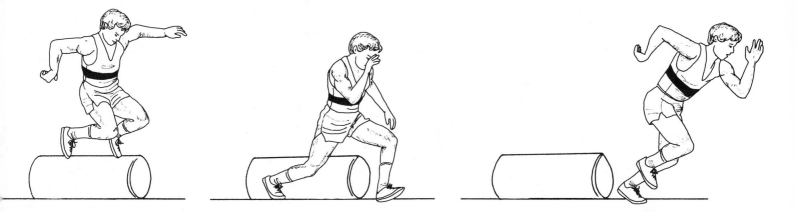

LEAPS

Drill: Quick Leap

A rather soft landing surface such as grass or a wrestling mat and a bench, stool, or box approximately 12 to 24 inches high are needed for the quick leap drill. The major muscle groups affected include the hip flexors, quadriceps, hamstrings, gluteals, lower back, and shoulder girdle. This exercise is useful in volleyball, football, basketball, platform diving, and weightlifting.

Starting position

With feet together, assume a semi-erect position facing the box (about 15 to 20 inches away). Keep the arms at the sides and slightly bent at the elbows.

Action sequence

Leap toward the box by exploding powerfully out of the starting position with the help of an energetic arm swing. While moving through the air, keep the knees high and forward of the hips, tucking the feet under the buttocks. Upon landing flat-footed on the box, assume a semi-squat position to absorb the shock and then immediately thrust forward again, this time extending and straightening the entire body. Finish by landing flat-footed on the ground with legs bent to act as a

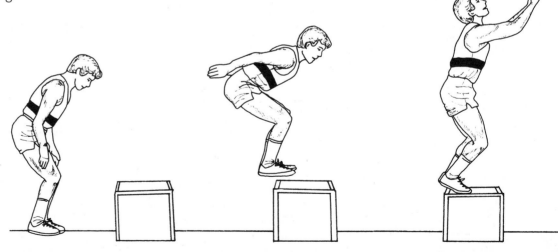

cushion. Make the initial jump to the box as quickly as possible with just enough height to reach the box. An-ticipate and concentrate on the second explosion from the box; stress a full extension of the body after leaping from the box. A variation of this exercise can be performed by landing on the box with only one foot, thus executing the leap with one driving leg.

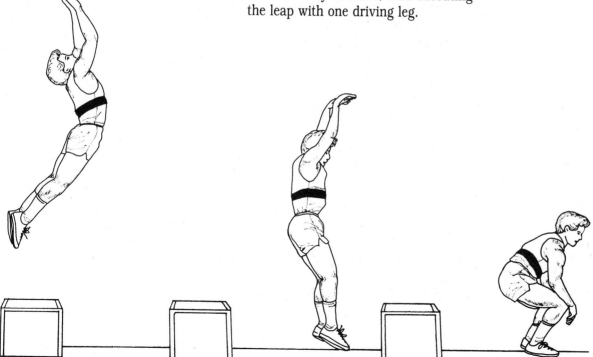

Drill: Depth Jump Leap

Two boxes or benches, one about 18 inches high and the other about 30 inches high, are required for this drill. Use a resilient landing surface such as grass or a wrestling mat. Major muscle groups employed in this exercise include quadriceps, hamstrings, gluteals, hip flexors, and gastrocnemius. This drill is very applicable to weightlifting, basketball, volleyball, ski jumping, and platform diving.

Starting position

Stand on the lower of the two boxes with arms at the sides; feet should be together and slightly off the edge as in the depth jump. The higher box is placed about 2 feet away in front of and facing the exerciser.

Action sequence

Begin by dropping off the lower box as in the depth jump, landing on the ground with both feet. Immediately jump onto the higher box, landing on both feet or on one foot, then drive upward and forward as intensely as possible, using the arms and a full exten-

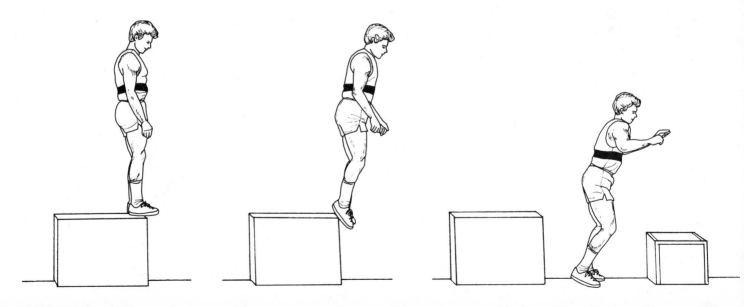

sion of the body. Complete the motion by landing on both feet with legs flexed to cushion the impact. Concentrate on a very quick, explosive depth jump, overcoming the force of landing and using the recoil to leap to the higher box. Think of driving hard off the higher box with the landing leg.

Three to 6 sets of leaps with each leg, resting about 1 minute between leaps, are suggested.

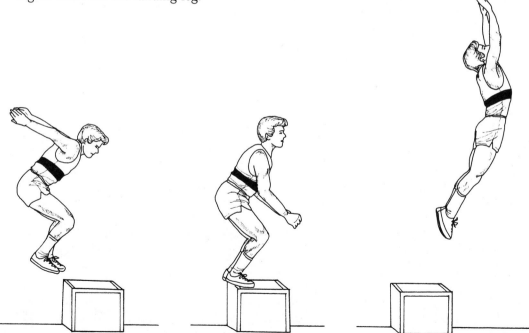

SKIPS

Drill: Skipping

Skipping, with full flexion of the leg, is an excellent drill for working the striding muscles: gluteals, gastrocnemius, quadriceps, hamstrings, and hip flexors. The muscles of the lower back, abdominals, and the shoulder girdle are also involved. Use a flat, semi-resilient surface for skipping. This is an excellent drill for high jumpers.

Starting position

Assume a relaxed standing position with one leg slightly forward of the other.

Action sequence

Driving off with the back leg, initiate a short skipping step, then with the opposite leg thrust the knee up to chest level; upon landing, repeat the action with the opposite leg. The pattern of right-right-step-left-left-step-right-right is executed. Obtain as much height and explosive power as possible after each short step (skip). Remember to drive the knee up hard and fast to generate maximal lift. Also, use the arms to initiate the lift after each skip. Concentrate on "hang-time" of the body and minimize the time the feet are in contact with the ground.

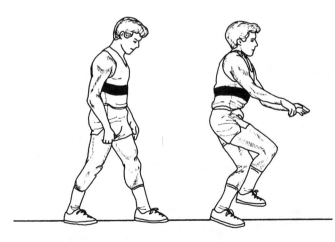

Three to 6 sets of 10 to 20 skips are
suggested; rest about 2 minutes
between sets.

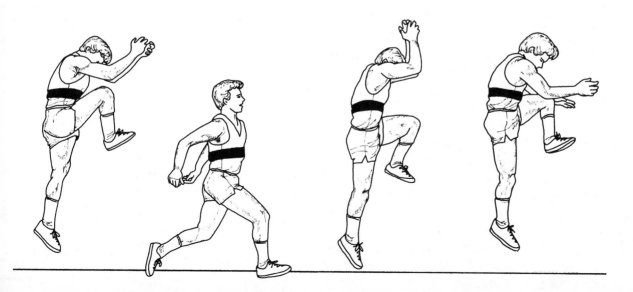

Drill: Box Skip

Two to 4 boxes in heights of 12 to 24 inches are needed for this exercise. The gluteals, gastrocnemius, quadriceps, hamstrings, hip flexors, muscles of the lower the back, and abdominals are all affected by this drill, which is especially applicable to basketball, Alpine skiing, and running events.

Starting position

Place the boxes in any order of height about 2 to 3 feet apart. Facing the first box from about 2 steps away, assume an upright stance with one leg slightly behind the other. Arms should be relaxed at the sides.

Action sequence

Drive off the back leg attempting to gain as much height with the knee as possible. Use the arms in an upward swinging motion to assist in the explosion. Immediately upon landing on the box, drive the other leg upward, gaining maximum height as before. Momentum from this action is used to leap from the first box. The ground landing between the first and second

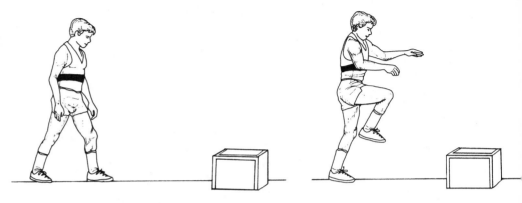

boxes is made with the same leg as the landing on the first box, thus the skip. Use the ground landing leg to drive toward the next box, now landing on the alternate leg. Continue the action sequence over the remaining boxes and concentrate on driving the knees upward with quickness and maximum force. Try to achieve maximum height with each explosive lift-off and think "hang-time."

Six sets of skips over 4 boxes with about 2 minutes rest between sets are suggested.

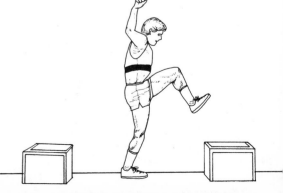

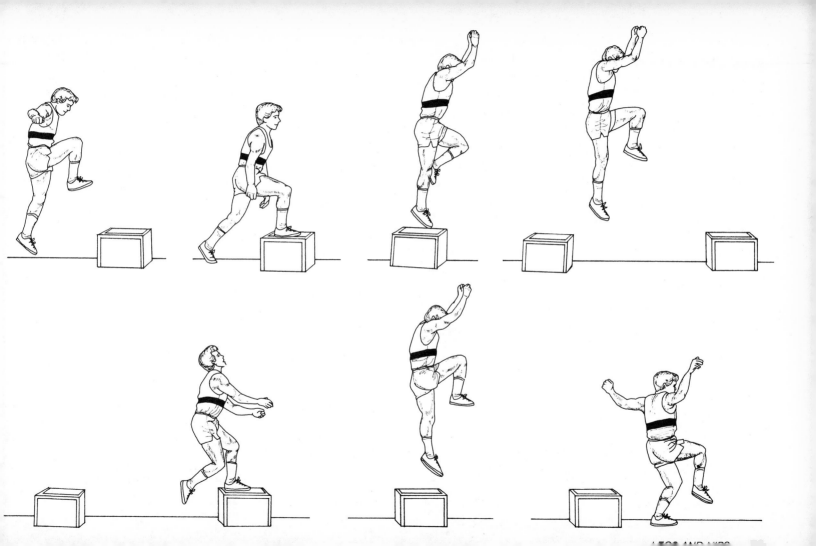

RICOCHETS

Drill: Incline Ricochet

For the ricochet, a set of stairs or stadium steps is required. Preferably the stairs should be solid, with no openings behind the treads for toes and feet to become entrapped. This exercise is designed for practicing reflexive quickness and is particularly well suited for football, basketball, soccer, baseball, tennis, and wrestling. The flexors of the lower leg and ankle stabilizers as well as the quadriceps, hamstrings, and thigh adductors and abductors are stressed.

Starting position

Face the bottom of the steps in a relaxed upright position with feet together and arms to the sides and cocked at the elbows.

Action sequence

Rapidly move up every step at the highest rate possible without tripping. Use the arms for balance, keeping thumbs up, and also for assisting in the explosion from step to step. Quickness is most important in this drill; anticipate hopping rapidly to each suc-ceeding step. Think of being light on the feet.

Variations of the ricochet can be accomplished by angling to the right or left of the steps or facing completely sideways. The ricochet can also be done one leg at a time to increase the load once the double-legged variations are mastered.

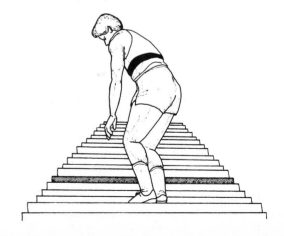

Perform 2 to 3 sets of 10 to 12 steps with a rest of about 2 minutes between sets. Jog slowly down the steps after each sequence.

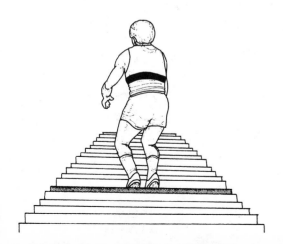
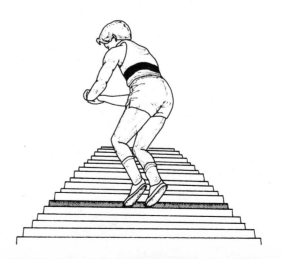

Drill: Decline Ricochet

This exercise is performed more safely on a grassy hill of about 2 to 4 degrees inclination. Quadriceps, gastrocnemius, extensors, and flexors of the lower legs and ankle as well as stabilizers of the knee are employed in this exercise. Furthermore, the neuromuscular systems involved in rapid, coordinated movement are trained.

Starting position

Assume a relaxed upright stance at the top of the hill facing down the fall line. Feet should be about shoulder-width apart.

Action sequence

Make a series of very short, rapid movements down the hill, rebounding from point to point as quickly as possible without falling forward. Hold the arms at the sides with elbows bent and keep thumbs up to help with balance. Concentrate on glancing off each contact point and being very light on the feet.

Perform 3 to 5 sets of 10 to 20 repetitions and rest about 1 minute between each set.

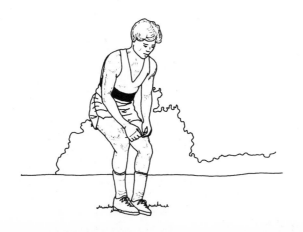
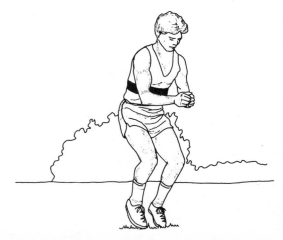

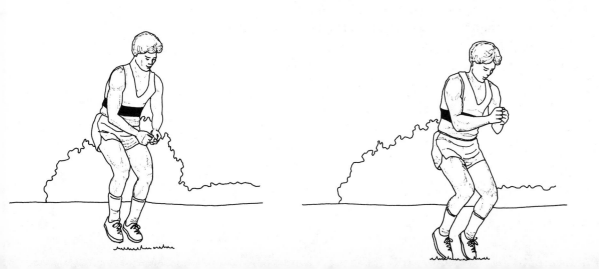

KIPS

Drill: Floor Kip

A soft flat surface such as a wrestling mat or thick grass is needed for this maneuver. The muscles of the hips, abdominals, lower back, shoulders, deltoids, arms, quadriceps, and hamstrings are all involved in doing kips. This exercise requires a high degree of coordination and explosive power in a total body effort, and is especially applicable to gymnastics, wrestling, weightlifting, and springboard diving.

Starting position

Assume a seated position with legs together and feet pointed.

Action sequence

Keeping legs extended and together, roll backward far enough so that the feet are brought past the head as in a reverse somersault. At the same time place the hands, palms down and fingers extended, on either side of the head. At this point the body will be in a cocked configuration. To initiate the power phase, rapidly extend the legs upward and forward while pushing against the floor with the hands. Extend the hips and arms forward now, flexing the legs and bringing them under the body in anticipation of the landing. Land in a semi-squat stance. Think of easing into a cocked position from the initial roll-back. Concentrate

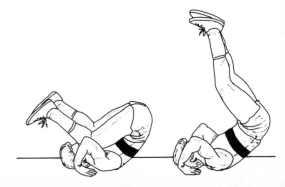

on exploding upward with the entire
body and, once airborne, remember to
shift the hips and arms quickly
forward.

Perform from 3 to 5 sets of 2 to 3
kips, resting about 2 minutes between
each set.

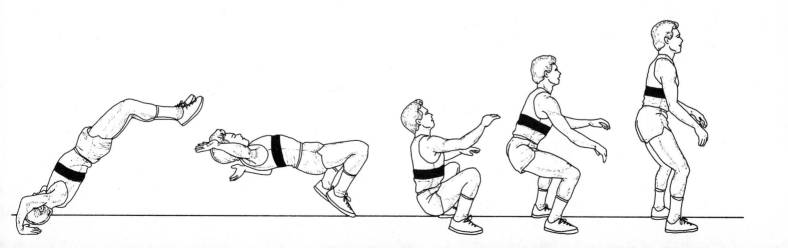

SWINGS

Drill: Horizontal Swing

A 15- to 30-pound dumbbell, swingbell, or other weighted object is required for this exercise, which involves muscles of the shoulders and arms as well as the posterior, lateral, and anterior trunk. The drill is excellent for developing torso power and is applicable to baseball, golf, hockey, shot-put and discus, football, and swimming.

Starting position

Feet and hips should be square with the body in a comfortable stance. With arms extended, hold the dumbbell at chest level with both hands at arm's length in front of the body; elbows should be slightly bent.

Action sequence

Initiate a torquing motion by pulling to one side with shoulder and arm. As momentum increases, begin to check the motion by pulling in the opposite direction with the other shoulder and arm. Begin the checking action before the torso has swung fully in one direction, that is, use the momentum in one direction as the load (cocking action) for eliciting a plyometric response in the other direction. Allow the work to

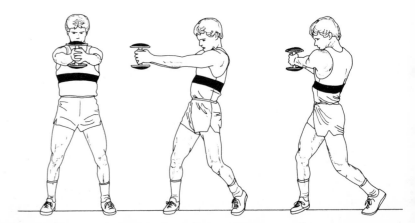

come from the shoulders and arms as well as the torso, using only minimal hip and leg involvement.

Perform 3 to 6 sets of 10 to 20 repetitions with approximately 1-minute rest periods between sets.

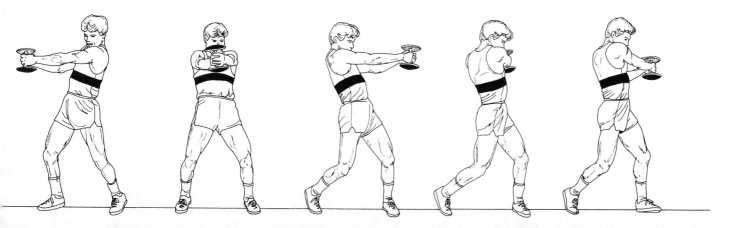

Drill: Vertical Swing

Use a dumbbell, swingbell, or similar object weighing about 15 to 30 pounds as in the horizontal swing. Shoulder, arm, lower back, chest, and anterior trunk muscles are all engaged in this movement. In addition to the athletic applications just mentioned for the horizontal swing, the vertical swing is quite beneficial for weightlifting, Nordic skiing, wrestling, volleyball, and swimming.

Starting position

Grasping the dumbbell with both hands, allow it to hang at arm's length between the outstretched legs. The back should be straight and the head should be up.

Action sequence

Keeping arms extended, swing the dumbbell first in an upward and then a downward motion. Resist the momentum of the dumbbell in one direction with a forceful braking effort to initiate movement in the opposite direction. Try to localize the workload

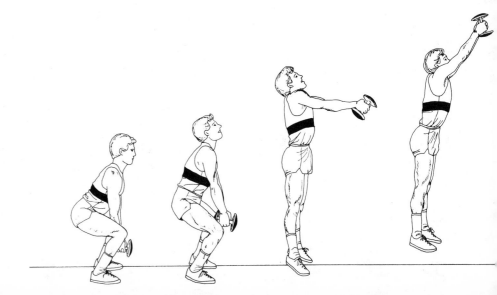

on the muscles of the shoulder girdle and upper back, minimizing involvement of hips and legs.

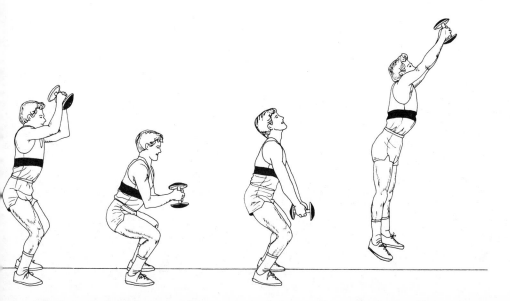

TWISTS

Drill:
Medicine Ball Twist/Toss

A 9- to 15-pound medicine ball is ideal for this exercise, which works the abdominals, latissimus, obliques, lower back, hips, biceps (arms), and pectoral muscles. Medicine ball twists are applicable in training for throwing and swinging.

Starting position

Cradle the ball next to the body at about waist level. Feet should be spaced slightly wider than shoulders.

Action sequence

Initiate the action by rapidly twisting the torso in the direction opposite the intended toss. Abruptly check the initial action with a quick and powerful twist in the opposite direction, releasing the ball after maximum torsion is reached. Concentrate on a rapid, reactive cocking action before twisting in the direction of the throw. Use the hips as well as the shoulders and arms.

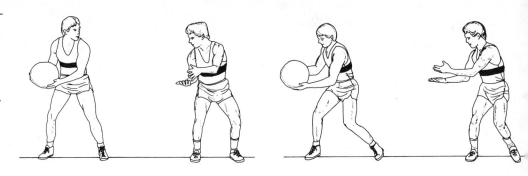

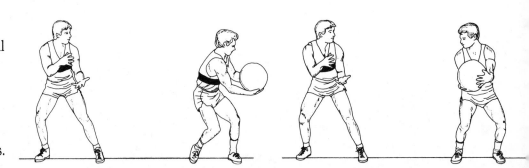

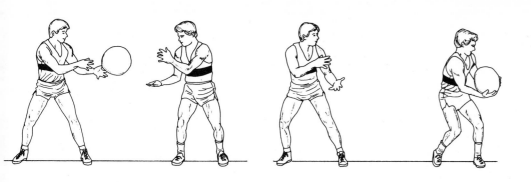

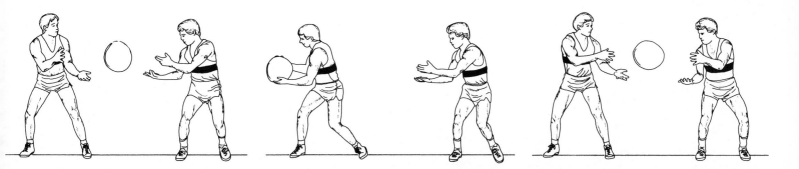

Drill: Bar Twist

A weighted bar of about 20 to 50 pounds is used in this drill. The movement is similar to the horizontal swing except that the bar twist is more concentrated on the trunk musculature with little active involvement of shoulders and arms. It is applicable to training for baseball, Nordic skiing, swimming, wrestling, golf, tennis, and most throwing actions.

Starting position

Standing upright, place the bar on the shoulders and hold it securely with both hands as far out from the center as possible. Feet should be slightly more than shoulder-width apart.

Action sequence

Twist the upper body in one direction, then before the torso is fully rotation. Repeat this sequence, actively driving the bar in one direction then the other. Think of using the muscles of the torso to accomplish the yielding and overcoming of the bar's momentum.

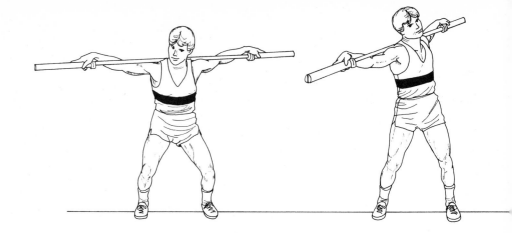

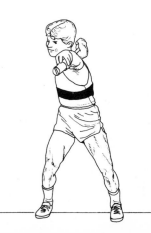

Perform about 20 to 30 repetitions for 3 to 5 sets; rest a minute between each set.

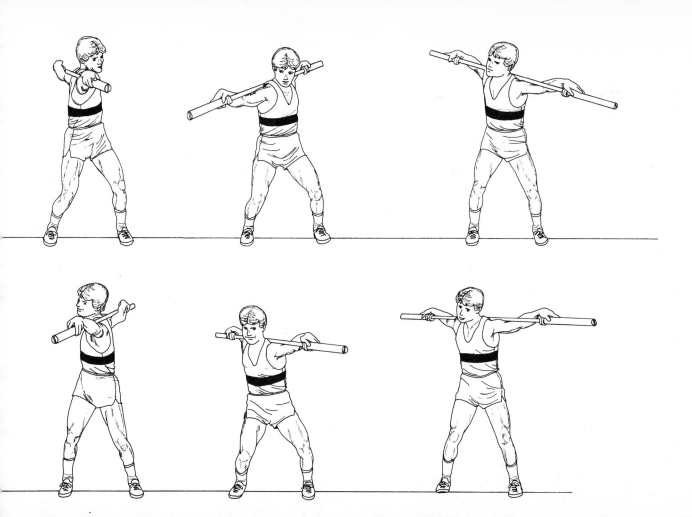

FLEXIONS

Drill:
Medicine Ball Sit-Up Throw

In this drill a 9- to 15-pound medicine ball is thrown between partners. The exercise directly stresses shoulders, arms, and abdominals and has wide application in sports such as wrestling, Nordic skiing, gymnastics, and football.

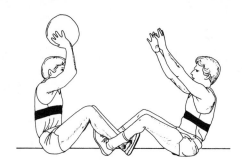
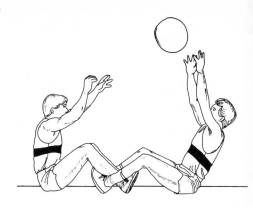

Starting position
Partners sit on the floor facing each other with feet interlocked. One partner holds the ball above the head while the other, anticipating the throw, holds the hands over the head to receive the ball.

Action sequence
The ball is thrown with a two-hand overhand action. Its momentum when caught by the other partner forces his or her torso to rock backward to absorb the shock. This backward motion is resisted with the abdominals and is also the cue to initiate the return toss of the ball. Concentrate on propelling the ball with the muscles of the trunk, not the arms and shoulders. Aim the toss to a point above your partner's head so that the arc of the throw is longer, producing greater momentum. Keep the arms extended overhead.

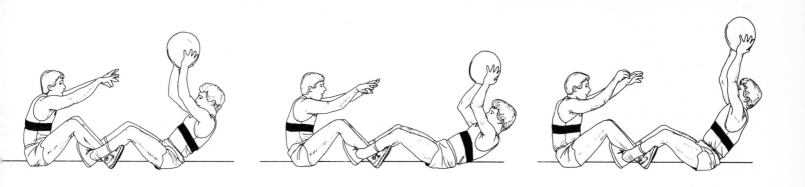

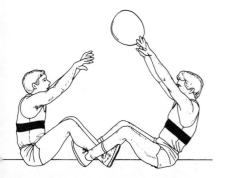

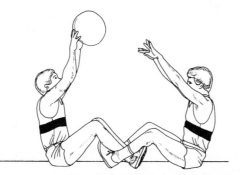

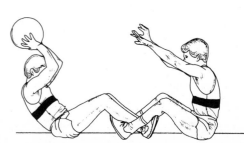

Drill:
Medicine Ball Leg Toss

Equipment for this maneuver includes a 9- to 16-pound medicine ball and horizontal bar, chin bar, or Swedish stall bars. This exercise requires full-body involvement affecting not only the abdominals and hip flexors but also the latissimus, arm, and shoulder muscles. It is applicable to weightlifting, soccer, high diving, football, and gymnastics.

Starting position

One partner hangs with both hands from an appropriate bar so that feet are just touching the ground. The other partner is several feet away, ready to roll the medicine ball.

Action sequence

The ball is rolled in the direction of the hanging partner. As the feet make contact with the ball, it is caught, its momentum checked with a forceful swing of the legs and flexion of the hips in the opposite direction. Concentrate on keeping the legs straight and using the hips to generate most of the

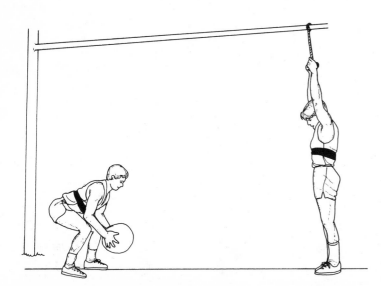

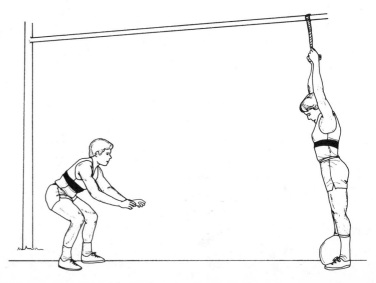

counterforce. The ball is retrieved by
the other partner and the sequence is
repeated.

Perform 2 to 4 sets of 8 to 12 repetitions, resting about 2 minutes between
sets.

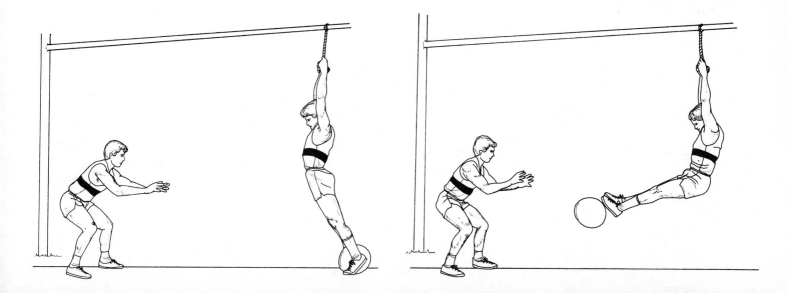

EXTENSIONS

Drill:
Medicine Ball Scoop Toss

A 9- to 15-pound medicine ball is required for this exercise, which involves lower back, hip flexors, shoulder girdle, arms, and quadriceps. This drill requires virtually a full-body power movement and is particularly applicable to weightlifting, football, volleyball, and wrestling.

Starting position

Assume a semi-squat stance. Place the ball between the legs, grasping it on either side with fingers spread. Arms should be extended, head held up, and back held straight.

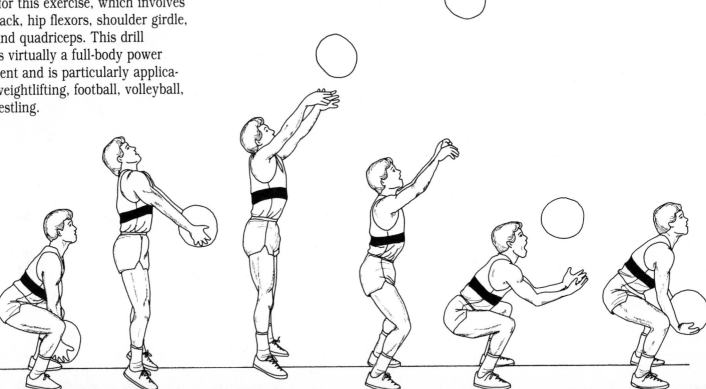

Action sequence

Begin by thrusting the hips forward and moving the shoulders backward while maintaining full extension of the arms. Scoop the ball upward, using the muscles of the shoulder girdle and arms as well as the back, hips, and legs. Catch the ball and place it again between the legs to repeat the motion. Concentrate on fully extending the body during the tossing phase.

Perform 3 to 6 sets of 8 to 10 repetitions; rest about 1 minute between sets.

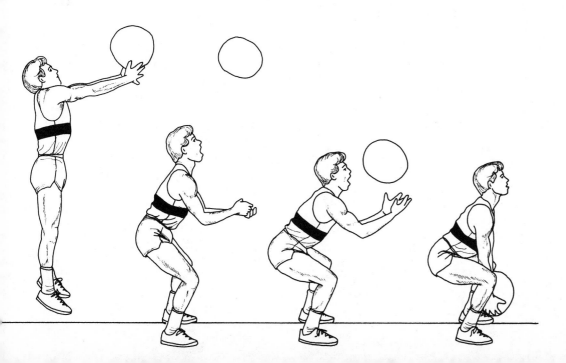

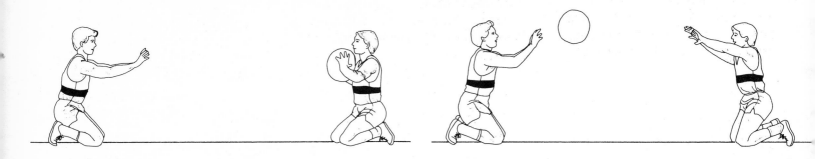

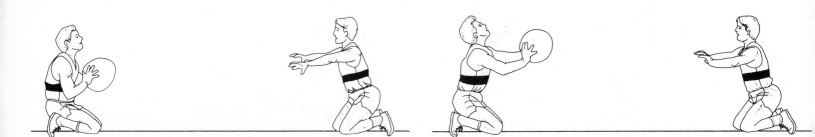

Chapter 7 UPPER BODY

PRESSES

Drill:
Medicine Ball Chest Pass

Use a 9- to 15-pound medicine ball for this exercise, which preferably is performed with a partner. The triceps, pectorals, latissimus, deltoids, and wrist and forearm muscles are engaged in this exercise. The movement is quite specific to the basketball chest pass, but is also beneficial in weight-lifting, wrestling, and shot-put.

Starting position

Partners stand or sit facing each other. One partner holds the ball at chest height with hands slightly behind the ball and arms flexed with the back of the hands touching the chest. The other partner anticipates the catch with arms extended horizontally at the chest.

Action sequence

The ball is pushed rapidly outward by one partner, extending arms to full length. The other partner checks the momentum of the ball and, before fully collapsing the arms, pushes outward in the opposite direction, passing it back with a full follow-through. The sequence is repeated back and forth in "catch" fashion.

Two to 4 sets of 20 to 30 repetitions with about 2 minutes rest between each set are recommended.

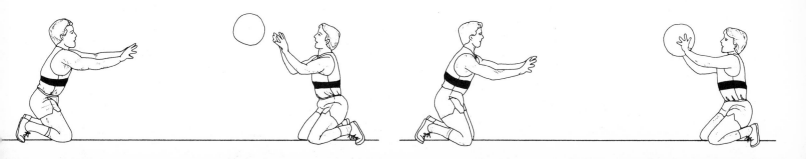

Drill: Heavy Bag Thrust

This exercise requires a heavy punching bag suspended from a rope or cable and involves the triceps, pectorals, deltoids, biceps (arms), trapezius, abdominals, external obliques, and hip extensor muscles. The drill is well suited for use by discus throwers, shotputters, and weightlifters as well as football and basketball players.

Starting position

Face the punching bag with legs in a semi-split position; the foot next to the bag is back. Place the inside hand chest high on the bag with fingers pointing upward; the elbow should be close to the body and the arm should be fully flexed.

Action sequence

Keeping the feet stationary and mainly using the torso, push the bag away from the body as rapidly as possible, extending the arm and shoulder fully. Catch the return flight of the bag with open hand and break the momentum using the trunk, arm, and shoulder muscles. Push the bag forward again before it reaches the original starting position. Concentrate on maintaining the same body stance throughout the entire drill. Switch sides and repeat, stressing quickness and explosiveness.

Perform 3 to 6 sets of 10 to 20 thrusts; rest about 2 minutes between sets.

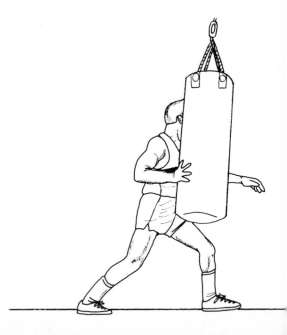

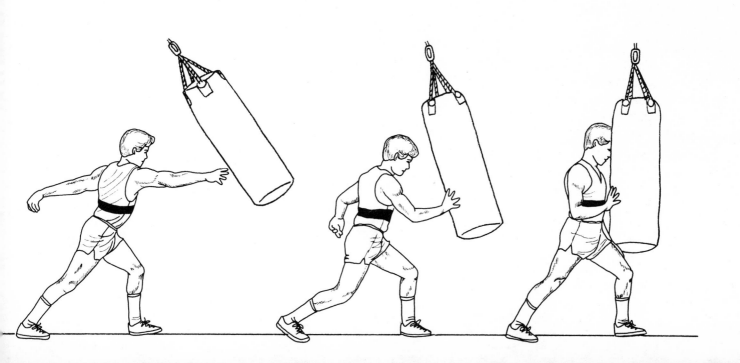

SWINGS

Drill: Dumbbell Arm Swings

Dumbbells or similar weighted handles of from 10 to 40 pounds are used in this drill, which employs shoulder and arm muscles and simulates the alternate arm movement of running and cross-country skiing.

Starting position

Hold the dumbbells firmly, one in each hand. Assume a comfortable stance with feet apart and hands at the sides. Keep the head straight and tilt the shoulders slightly forward.

Action sequence

Drive one arm upward to a point just above the head while driving the other arm backward behind the body. Before each arm reaches maximum stretch, check the momentum by initiating motion in the opposite direction. Continue this alternating sequence for 20 to 30 swings. A variation of this basic pattern is performed by holding the dumbbells in a half-flexed position with the arms. Such "running curls" simulate more closely the arm and shoulder motion executed while sprinting. In running curls, try to accomplish quick, rapid swings, keeping the elbows close to the body.

Perform 2 to 4 sets with a 2-minute rest between each set.

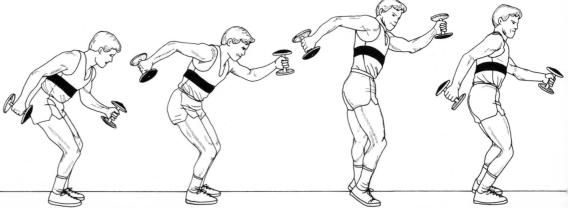

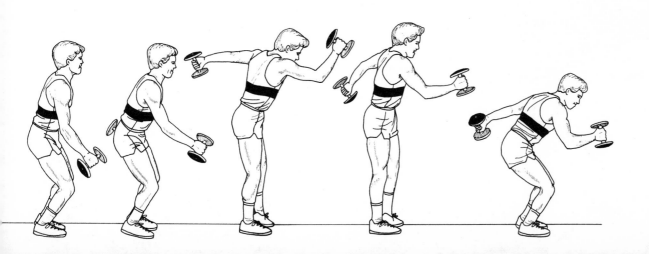

Drill: Heavy Bag Stroke

A heavy punching bag suspended from a rope or cable is required. This drill simulates the motion often associated with a tennis stroke but is also applicable for training in baseball, discus, and javelin. It works the twisting muscles of the trunk as well as the muscles of the arms and shoulders.

Starting position

Assume an upright stance next to the heavy bag. Feet should be slightly more than shoulder-width apart. With arm extended, rest the forearm across the bag at chest height.

Action sequence

Begin by twisting at the waist, keeping the arm extended and pushing the bag with the forearm. Continue the action until the bag is moved away from the body. Catch the bag upon its return flight with the same position of the arm that was used in initiating the movement. Check the momentum of the bag with the same muscle groups used to initially propel it and then powerfully reapply force in the opposite direction. Remember to follow through, rotating at the waist with each push.

Perform 2 to 4 sets of 10 to 20 strokes on each arm.

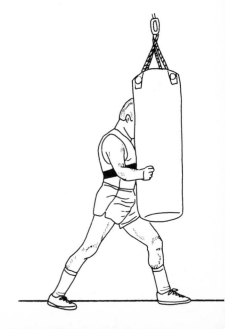

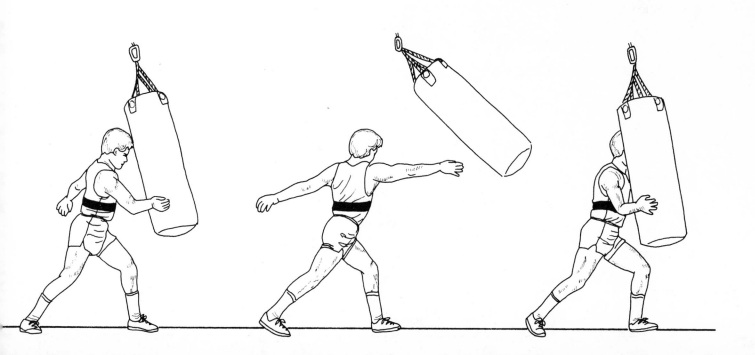

THROWS

Drill: Medicine Ball Throw

Use a 9- to 16-pound medicine ball for this drill. Shoulder, arm, chest, and trunk muscles are involved in a motion specific to the soccer throw but also applicable to Nordic skiing, basketball, wrestling, and volleyball.

Starting position

Assume a kneeling position with knees positioned at about shoulder-width. Hold the ball firmly on the sides and slightly back, positioning it behind the head with arms bent.

Action sequence

Slowly lean back with the ball positioned behind the head; as the momentum of this motion builds, rapidly check it with a powerful forward flexion of the torso. Follow through by throwing the ball out as far as possible. Concentrate on thrusting

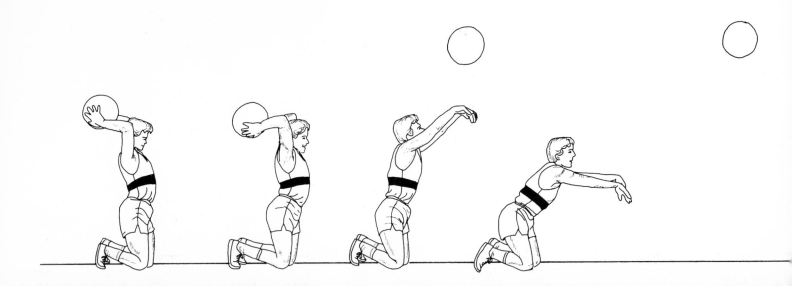

the arms forward from the shoulders
and chest.

Perform 3 to 6 sets of 10 to 20
throws; rest about 2 minutes between
sets.

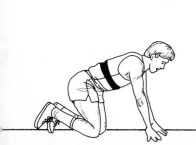
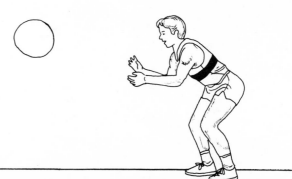

Appendix A
PHYSIOLOGICAL BASIS
FOR PLYOMETRIC EXERCISES

In this appendix you can learn more about how scientists think plyometric training works. We will examine in some detail the neuromuscular elements involved and why plyometric exercises have been found successful in training for explosive power. Although quite technical, this discussion will help you understand and appreciate the intricate nature of what takes place at the neuromuscular level.

Remember, plyometric movement is believed to be based on the reflex contraction of muscle fibers resulting from the rapid loading (and thus stretching) of these same muscle fibers. The primary sensory receptor responsible for detecting rapid elongation of muscle fibers is the muscle spindle, which is capable of responding to both the magnitude and rate of change in length of muscle fibers. Another type of stretch receptor, the Golgi tendon organ, is located in the tendons and responds to excessive tension as a result of powerful contractions and/or stretching of the muscle. Of the two, the muscle spindle is probably more important to plyometrics. Both of these sensory receptors function at the reflex level. Although no sensory perception is associated with either, both transmit large amounts of information to the brain (e.g., cerebellum and cerebral cortex) via the spinal cord and thus are very important elements in overall motor control by the central nervous system.

The structure of the muscle spindle, shown on page 112 (top), reveals some interesting features that shed light into how these mechanoreceptors may function during plyometric movement. Each muscle spindle comprises several specially adapted muscle fibers (about 1 cm long) referred to as intrafusal fibers. The central portions of intrafusal fibers lack the ability to contract, containing neither of the contractile proteins actin and myosin. However, the end portions of the intrafusals, which attach to the connective sheaths of the skeletal muscle fibers, do contain actin and myosin and thus are capable of contraction. Two different types of intrafusal fibers are discernible (see page 112, bottom). Some intrafusals have large central bulges filled with cell nuclei, the so-called nuclear bag fibers. Others are narrower and

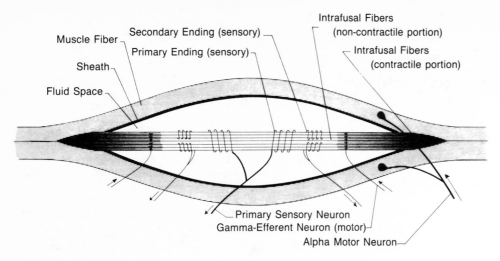

Muscle Fiber
Secondary Ending (sensory)
Primary Ending (sensory)
Sheath
Fluid Space
Intrafusal Fibers (non-contractile portion)
Intrafusal Fibers (contractile portion)
Primary Sensory Neuron
Gamma-Efferent Neuron (motor)
Alpha Motor Neuron

contain single chains of cell nuclei at their centers. These are the so-called nuclear chain fibers. Differences in the function of these two types of intra-fusals will be discussed shortly.

Innervation of the muscle spindle is complex; both sensory and motor nerves are involved. The main sensory innervation is located at the centers of the nuclear bag intrafusal fibers. These nerve endings form a coil-like structure (annulospiral ending) around the intra-

fusals and are the actual receptors for detecting changes in length of the intrafusals. Because the intrafusals are

firmly attached at their ends to the cell walls of the skeletal muscle fibers, any change in length of the latter results in a change in length of the intrafusals and thus a movement in the coil-like ending of the sensory receptor.

In addition to the primary ending coiled around the centers of the nuclear bag intrafusal fibers, the primary sensory neuron also sends out branches that wind around the centers of the nuclear chain intrafusals. The sensory neurons associated with the primary receptors are very large in diameter (about 17 microns) and are capable of transmitting nervous impulses to the spinal cord and brain at velocities of about 100 meters per

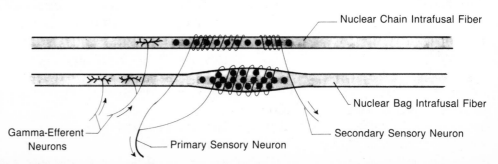

Nuclear Chain Intrafusal Fiber
Nuclear Bag Intrafusal Fiber
Secondary Sensory Neuron
Gamma-Efferent Neurons
Primary Sensory Neuron

second, which is about as fast as any nerve fibers in the body are capable of doing.

In addition to the annulospiral endings of the primary receptors, two other sensory endings—located one on either side of the annulospiral ending—innervate the muscle spindles. However, these secondary receptors are associated only with the noncontractile portions of the nuclear chain intrafusals, encircling them in a manner similar to that of the annulospiral ending of the primary receptor. The afferent neurons in the secondary receptor endings are much smaller in diameter (about 8 microns) than the neurons of the primary receptors and thus are capable of transmitting nervous impulses to the spinal cord at a velocity of about 50 meters per second.

Innervating the contractile ends of both nuclear chain and nuclear bag intrafusal fibers are efferent (motor) neurons from the spinal cord. The motor neurons are part of the gamma-efferent system and not associated with the alpha motor neurons that innervate the skeletal muscle fibers themselves. Some of the gamma-efferents innervate the nuclear chain intrafusals and others innervate the nuclear bag intrafusals.

From the description of the structure and innervation of the muscle spindle so far, it should be apparent that the primary as well as the secondary receptors can be activated in different ways. Because the ends of the intrafusal fibers, around which the primary receptor endings (annulospiral endings) are coiled, are attached to the skeletal muscle fibers, any lengthening of the latter (e.g., in rapid loading during athletic movement) will cause a stretching of the intrafusals and in turn the coiled endings of the primary receptors. The uncoiling of the annulospiral ending initiates a burst of nervous impulses sent to the spinal cord via the afferent sensory neurons. The contractile ends of the intrafusals are innervated by the gamma-efferent motor neurons; stimulation of the intrafusals in this manner can cause them to contract, stretching their central portions and in turn activating the primary receptors. This can occur even though the skeletal muscle fibers themselves (to which the intrafusals are attached) remain unstretched.

In terms of overall function, the muscle spindle is capable of emitting two types of responses (Guyton, 1981), static and dynamic. A "static" response may occur when the intrafusal fibers are slowly stretched, resulting from a gradual stretching of the skeletal muscle fibers or perhaps from direct stimulation of the intrafusals by the gamma-efferent system. In either case both the primary and secondary coiled receptors are slowly pulled apart, emitting a continuous, low-level stream of nervous impulses. As the magnitude of stretching increases, the rate of emission of nervous impulses also increases. This static response can continue for several minutes, as long as the skeletal muscle fibers remain stretched.

A property of all sensory receptors is their ability to adapt after some period of continuous stimulation. At first application of the stimulus, the response of the sensory receptor may be very high; as the application of the stimulus continues at the same level of intensity the response tends to drop off. In some sensory receptors such as pressure receptors of the skin, the adaptation is rapid and complete in less than a second, while in others such as the muscle spindles, the initial rate of adaptation may be very slow and complete adaptation may not be achieved even after several minutes. Muscle spindles and other such slowly adapting mechanoreceptors are thus capable of transmitting information about the state of contraction of the muscles and orientation of the limbs to the higher central nervous system centers, thus aiding the brain in overall motor control.

In the "dynamic" response of the muscle spindle, the primary receptor is activated by a rapid change in length of the intrafusal fiber around which it is coiled. When this happens, the primary receptor sends many impulses to the spinal cord. The important variable in the dynamic response appears to be the abruptness or rapidity with which the stretching occurs, not necessarily the degree of stretching. The dynamic response ceases almost as quickly as it is initiated, after which the muscle spindle resumes its static level of discharge.

This dynamic response of the muscle spindle is believed to be the important functional element of plyometric movement. Because the primary receptors are associated with the nuclear bag intrafusals, the latter are also considered to be associated in the detection of rapid stretching of the muscle. The nuclear chain intrafusals have both primary and secondary receptor innervation and are thus believed to be involved primarily with slow stretching (static response).

Just as the two types of intrafusal fibers can be functionally differentiated into those associated with the static response and those associated with the dynamic response, so can the motor neurons of the gamma-efferents. Apparently there are gamma-efferents that excite the nuclear bag intrafusals and are therefore important in controlling the dynamic response, and other gamma-efferents that stimulate the nuclear chain intrafusals and are therefore important in controlling the static response. The gamma-efferent system of the muscle spindle can thus function to increase or decrease the thresholds of response to stretching of both types of intrafusals. When the dynamic gamma-efferents are stimulated, the nuclear bag intrafusals are prestretched, allowing for even the smallest degree of external stretching of the skeletal muscle fiber to stimulate the primary receptor. Contractile stimulation of the nuclear chain intrafusals by the gamma-efferents increases the output level of the static response.

The main function of the muscle spindle is to elicit the so-called stretch or myotatic reflex, which is considered the neuromuscular process that typifies the action basis of plyometrics. Whenever the muscle fibers are rapidly loaded by outside forces, causing an abrupt stretching, the lengthening of the fibers is detected by the muscle spindle, eliciting this dynamic response. A large burst of impulses is sent to the spinal cord via the afferent neuron of the primary receptor. In the spinal cord the afferent neuron synapses directly with an alpha motor neuron, sending powerful impulses back to the skeletal muscle fibers and causing them to contract, thus overcoming the external forces.

The stretch reflex may also occur as a slower response. If the muscle is stretched gradually, thus stretching the nuclear chain intrafusals which function during the static response of the muscle spindle, then a slower, continuous transmission of impulses is sent to the spinal cord via appropriate afferent neurons; these synapse with alpha motor neurons, stimulating

lower intensity contraction of the skeletal muscle fibers. This may continue for several minutes as opposed to the dynamic stretch reflex, which usually is over in less than a second.

Plyometric exercises require that a rapid loading (eccentric or yielding phase) of the muscles be accomplished just prior to the contraction phase of these muscles. In the depth jump, for example, the exerciser drops from an elevated platform; as soon as the feet make contact with the ground the legs begin to bend under the increased load of g-forces (kinetic energy) developed by falling. The degree to which the legs bend upon impact is determined largely by the activity level of the muscle spindle reflex. For instance, if the gamma-efferents responsible for controlling the static level of the muscle spindle are highly active, so that the static reflex is at an elevated level, even a slight lengthening of the quadriceps (and therefore the muscle spindles of the quadriceps) will cause a very strong contraction of these

muscles through the dynamic stretch reflex.

The influence of the gamma-efferent stimulation on the magnitude and intensity of the dynamic stretch reflex is very important. An understanding of this relationship is essential in conceptualizing the nature of plyometric training. If in the example of the depth jump the level of gamma-static efferent stimulation to the muscle spindles of the quadriceps were very low, then the sensitivity of the spindle to sudden stretching would be depressed and the effectiveness of the dynamic stretch reflex would be almost nil. Consequently, the jump (contraction, overcoming) phase of the exercise could not be performed in a powerful manner. Conversely, if the gamma-static efferents were firing at a high rate during the exercise, then the threshold for eliciting the dynamic stretch reflex would be greatly lowered; the slightest stretching of the quadriceps upon landing would cause a potent dynamic stretch reflex to occur.

Many of the plyometric exercises described in Part III require phases in which one muscle group or another is held in an isometric position just prior to the explosive (concentric or overcoming) phase. The instantaneous reflex resistance that attempts to prevent the limb from being moved rapidly from its assumed isometric position is the result of the dynamic stretch or load reflex. Through volitional pathways controlled by higher centers of the brain, the sensitivity of the load reflex can be changed by altering the intensity of the gamma-static stimulation of the muscle spindle.

The role of the gamma-efferent system in dampening or enhancing the degree of responsiveness of the muscle spindles is also extremely important in overall motor control. Some body movements must be executed in a smooth and continuous manner, for example, the dance-like and rhythmic motions of katas in the martial arts. In the execution of such nonexplosive movements, the gamma-efferents function to dampen the responsiveness of the muscle spindle to changes in length of the muscles being used. However, when the requirement is to move the limbs very quickly and powerfully in response to an instantaneous change in resistive input, as in plyometrics, then dampening by the gamma-efferent system is greatly lowered.

Conscious control of the reactivity levels of the muscle spindles is possible through the gamma-efferent system. Thus, one may concentrate on performing muscular movements that are either smooth and continuous or explosive and powerful. Centers in the brain known to be associated with control of the gamma-efferent system are regions of the brain stem, cerebellum, and the cerebral cortex itself. The exact mechanisms involved in this control have yet to be elucidated. Suffice it to say there are very complex input and feedback loops between the muscle spindles and these areas in the control of muscle contraction, as well as overall motor control.

Plyometric training works within the context of these intricate and complex neural mechanisms. Presumably, as a result of plyometric training, changes occur at both muscular and neural levels that facilitate and enhance the performance of more rapid and powerful movement skills.

Also involved in the control of muscular contraction is the Golgi tendon organ. This mechanoreceptor is located in the tendon itself and is stimulated by tensile forces generated by the contraction of muscle fibers to which it is attached. It responds maximally to sudden increases in tension and transmits a lower, more continuous level of impulses when tension is decreased.

The Golgi tendon reflex occurs when muscle tension is increased; signals transmitted to the spinal cord cause an inhibitory (negative feedback) response to the contracted muscle, thus preventing an inordinate amount of tension from developing in the muscle. The

Golgi tendon organ is thought to be a protective device, preventing tearing of the muscle and/or tendon under extreme conditions, but it may also work in concert with the muscle spindle reflex for achieving overall control of muscle contraction and body movement.

The contractile elements of the muscles are the muscle fibers. Certain parts of muscles are noncontractile: the ends of the muscle fiber sheaths where they connect to the tendons, the cross-membranes of the muscle fibers, and the tendons. Together the noncontractile portions of muscles constitute what is known as the series elastic component. Recent evidence (Robertson, 1984) suggests that the contractile machinery of the muscle fibers themselves may contribute to the series elastic component.

When a muscle contracts, the structures of the series elastic component stretch as much as 3 to 5% of the muscle fiber length. An analogous action is that of a nylon rope under increased tension; it stretches some portion of its total length before becoming completely taut. The stretching of the series elastic component during muscle contraction produces an elastic potential energy similar to that of a loaded spring or a drawn bow. When this energy is released, it augments to some degree the energy of contraction generated by the muscle fibers.

In plyometric movements during the eccentric or yielding phase, when the muscle is being rapidly stretched, the series elastic component is also stretched, thus storing a portion of the load force in the form of elastic potential energy. The recovery of the stored elastic energy occurs during the concentric or overcoming phase of muscle contraction, which is triggered by the myotatic reflex.

Appendix B
PLYOMETRIC TESTING PROCEDURES

TEST #1:
VERTICAL JUMP

(a) The athlete stands flat-footed next to a wall or pole, and with chalked fingers or an attached piece of tape he or she reaches up and places a mark at the highest point possible.

(b) Remaining in the same place, the athlete will summon all of the forces possible and jump upward off both legs, touching the wall at the highest point of the jump.

(c) Again the athlete should have tape or chalk on the fingers in order to make a substantial mark at the two points of emphasis.

(d) The distance between the two marks is the athlete's jump reach height. The highest (jumping) mark will be the criteria for the depth jump test.

(e) Take the best of three such jump

trials, allowing 30 seconds to a minute of rest between each trial to allow the muscle system to recuperate.

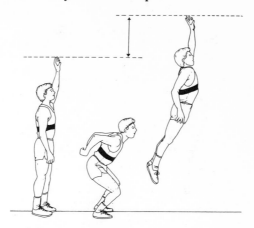

TEST #2:
DEPTH JUMP
HEIGHTS

(a) Using boxes of different heights or a stair-step apparatus, have the athlete

drop off from levels between 12 and 42 inches onto grass or a firm but resilient mat.

(b) Upon landing, the athlete should immediately jump upward in an attempt to reach or surpass the mark placed on the wall during the vertical jump test.

(c) The athlete should continue to move up in the height of each drop un-

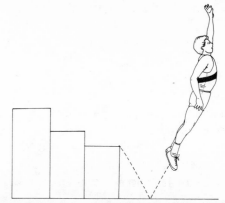

til he or she can no longer attain the same jump height as in the vertical jump.

(d) The point of the depth or drop height when maximum vertical jump (rebound) height was attained is the approximate height to train for in this type of plyometric exercise.

(e) Allow approximately 1 minute of rest between each trial so that the muscle systems can recover.

TEST #3:
BOX JUMP TEST

(a) Have the athlete stand directly in front of a box, sturdy table, or stair-step apparatus, the top height of which should be approximately mid-thigh level.

(b) Standing flat-footed and approximately an arm's length away, the athlete should summon all of the forces possible and jump up onto the top of the box or table.

(c) After each successful attempt, raise

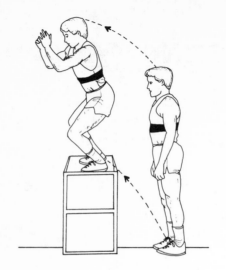

the height of the platform until the athlete finds it very difficult or impossible to jump up on it.

(d) Have the athlete use his or her hands when unable to make the attempt, as to catch, brace, or push away, and therefore to avoid falling on the box or table. Position mats all around the platform and always have spotters available to help the subject if an attempt fails.

TEST #4:
MEDICINE BALL PASS

(a) The athlete sits in a straight-back chair and is strapped in securely with a belt or waist harness.

(b) With a medicine ball of 9, 12, or 15 pounds, the athlete performs a chest pass, applying all the forces possible to the put.

(c) The distance from the chair to the ball's landing point determines how heavy a ball to use for such exercises.

(d) Any passes under approximately 10 to 12 feet in length indicate a need for training with a lighter medicine ball.

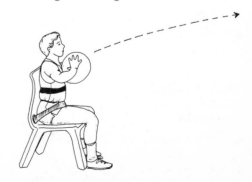

Appendix C
SPECIFICATIONS FOR BUILDING APPARATUS

JUMPING BOX

Materials

2 —2" x 4" x 48" boards for top
2 —2" x 4" x 16" boards for top
4 —2" x 4" x 12" studs for braces*
1 —16" x 48" x ¼" sheet plywood
2 —12" x 48" x ¼" sheet plywood*
2 —12" x 16" x ¼" sheet plywood*
46—1" wood screws for attaching plywood boards (3 per side and 3-5 per side on the top)

Encase all edges and corners with wood or aluminum molding (light gauge). Use #8 nails for brace connections.

*Note: The height of the box can vary. It can be 8", 12", 18", or 24".

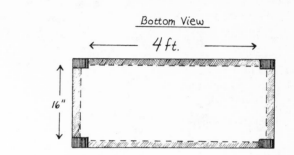

Bottom View

4 ft.

16"

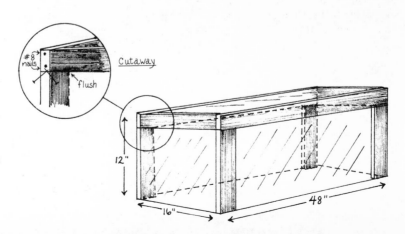

#8 nails

flush

Cutaway

12"

48"

16"

ANGLE BOX

Materials

4 —2" x 4" x 5' long boards for frame
and doubled for weight
3 —2" x 4" x 7" middle braces
2 —2" x 4" x 12" end boards
2 —2" x 4" x 13" end boards
2 —2" x 4" x 11" mid boards
6 —½" x 15" x ¼" plywood boards
36—1" wood screws for top platform
Use #8 nails for brace connections.

Note: The precise angles of this box are not
crucial. The importance lies in that each angle
is slightly different from the other three.

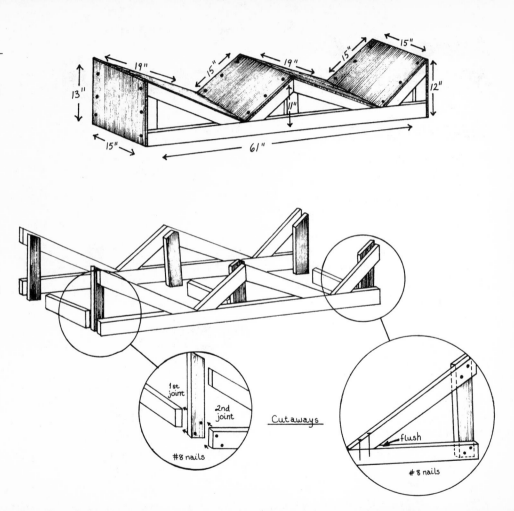

ANGLE BOARD

Materials

5 —½" x 12" x [*] plywood boards
    (per box)
28—wood dowels or screws for
    assembling each box

*Note: Sizes of boards differ in height and
top length according to box size desired.

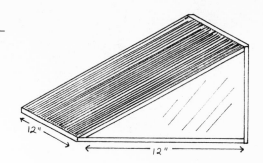

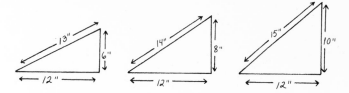

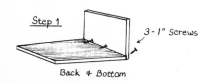

Step 1

3 - 1" Screws

Back & Bottom

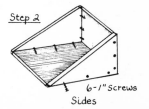

Step 2

6 - 1" Screws

Sides

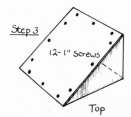

Step 3

12 - 1" Screws

Top

REFERENCES

Bosco, C., & Komi, P.V. (1979). Mechanical characteristics and fiber composition of human leg extensor muscles. *European Journal of Applied Physiology, 41*, 275-284.

Bosco, C., & Komi, P.V. (1981). Potentiation of the mechanical behavior of the human skeletal muscle through prestretching. *Acta Physiologica Scandinavica, 106*, 467-472.

Chu, D. (1983). Plyometrics: The link between strength and speed. *National Strength and Conditioning Association Journal, 5*, 20.

Chu, D. (1984). Plyometric exercise. *National Strength and Conditioning Association Journal, 5*, 26.

Costello, F. (1984). Using weight training and plyometrics to increase explosive power for football. *National Strength and Conditioning Association Journal, 6*(2), 22-25.

Gambetta, V. (1981). Plyometric training. In V. Gambetta (Ed.), *Track and field coaching manual* (pp. 58-59). West Point, NY: Leisure Press.

Guyton, A.C. (1981). *Textbook of medical physiology*. Philadelphia: W.B. Saunders.

Landis, D. (1983). Big skinny kids. *National Strength and Conditioning Association Journal, 5*, 26-29.

McArdle, W., Katch, F.I., & Katch, V.L. (1981). *Exercise physiology, energy, nutrition and human performance*. Philadelphia: Lea & Febiger.

McFarlane, B. (1982). Jumping exercises. *Track & Field Quarterly Review, 82*(4), 54-55.

Robertson, R.N. (1984). Compliance characteristics of human muscle during dynamic and static loading conditions (abstract). Clinical Symposium. *Medicine and Science in Sports and Exercise, 16*, 186.

Sinclair, A. (1981). A reaction to depth jumping. *Sports Coach, 5*(2), 24-25.

Tansley, J. (1980). *The flop book*. Santa Monica, CA: Peterson Lithograph.

Valik, B. (1966). Strength preparation of young track and fielders. Physical Culture in School, 4:28. In *Yessis Translation Review* (1967) **2**, 56-60.

Veroshanski, Y. (1966). Perspectives in the improvement of speed-strength preparation of jumpers. Track and Field 9:11. In *Yessis Review of Soviet Physical Education and Sports* (1969), **4**, 28-34.

Veroshanski, Y. (1967). Are depth jumps useful? Track and Field 12:9. In *Yessis Review of Soviet Physical Education and Sports* (1968), **3**, 75.

Veroshanski, Y., & Chernousov, G. (1974). Jumps in the training of a sprinter. Track and Field **9**:16. In *Review of Soviet Physical Education and Sports* (1974), **9**, 62-66.

Wilt, F., & Ecker, T. (1970). *International Track and Field Coaching Encyclopedia.* West Nyack, NY: Parker Publ.

ABOUT THE AUTHORS

Authors James Radcliffe and Robert Farentinos combine their experience and knowledge to make *Plyometrics* a unique blend of theory and application.

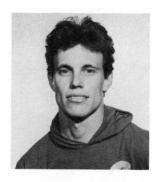

Jim Radcliffe received a bachelor's degree in physical education at Pacific University. Presently a graduate student at the University of Colorado, Jim has had nearly 10 years of practical experience in plyometric training. He taught and coached at the high school level and has been a coaching consultant for schools in the Boulder area. Many of the drills in the book originated through Radcliffe's plyometric research and coaching. He has also published the *Plyometrics Methods Notebook*.

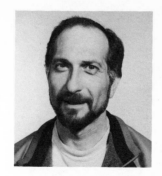

With a PhD in biology from the University of Colorado and 17 years of teaching experience in anatomy and physiology, Dr. Farentinos uses his wide-ranging knowledge to explain the physiology behind plyometric conditioning. Dr. Farentinos also has an extensive background in muscular conditioning through his experience as a competitive weightlifter and as a member of the U.S. Marathon Ski Team. Presently, he manages an athletic training, fitness-conditioning complex that specializes in applying the fundamentals of exercise physiology and anatomy to help improve athletic performance. Through his work, Dr. Farentinos has consulted with the U.S. cycling, weightlifting, and ski teams.

ANOTHER "POWERFUL" TRAINING TOOL FROM HUMAN KINETICS

PLYOMETRICS: EXPLOSIVE POWER TRAINING FOR EVERY SPORT (50-MINUTE VIDEOTAPE)

Now that you've read about plyometrics, perfect your technique with this dynamic videotape from the authors of *Plyometrics*. You'll find detailed demonstrations and explanations of each exercise, so you'll never have to second guess about proper techniques. And, you'll also learn about the applications of plyometrics to various sports, as well as the scientific principles behind them. Complete with highlights from noted sports coaches and experts like Dr. Ed Burke of the U.S. Cycling Federation, and Don Nielsen and Pat Ahern of the U.S. Ski Team, this videotape is an ideal training tool for coaching staff and athletes, and an excellent companion to *Plyometrics: Explosive Power Training (Second Edition)*.

Item MPLY0022 • ½" VHS Video • $125
Item MPLY0023 • ¾" U-matic • $135
Item MPLY0024 • ½" Beta Video • $125

Human Kinetics Publishers, Inc. • **Box 5076** • **Dept. 469** • *Champaign, IL 61820*